KT-413-090

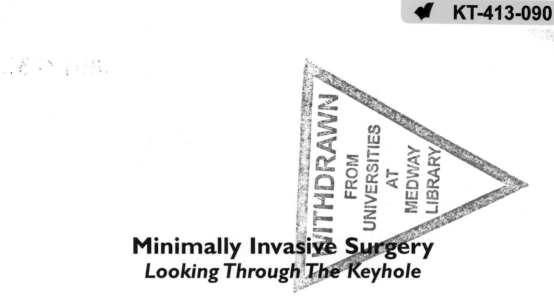

WITHDRAWN FROM UNIVERSITIES AT MEDWAY LIBRARY

Minimally Invasive Surgery
Looking Through The Keyhole

Edited by
Hitendra Patel and Jean Joseph

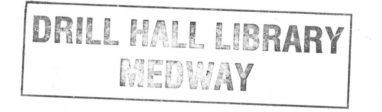

DRILL HALL LIBRARY
MEDWAY

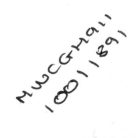

MWCGH91
1001189)

Other titles available

Urological Oncology: A day-to-day guide for the non-specialist
Edited by HRH Patel

8017232

Minimally Invasive Surgery
Looking Through The Keyhole

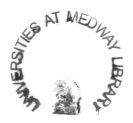

UNIVERSITIES AT MEDWAY LIBRARY

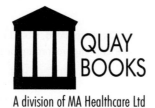

QUAY
BOOKS

A division of MA Healthcare Ltd

Quay Books Division, MA Healthcare Ltd, St Jude's Church, Dulwich Road, London SE24 0PB

British Library Cataloguing-in-Publication Data
A catalogue record is available for this book

© MA Healthcare Limited 2006
ISBN 1856422968

All rights reserved. No part of this publication may be reproduced, stored in a retrieval system or transmitted in any form or by any means, electronic, mechanical, photocopying, recording or otherwise, without prior permission from the publishers

Printed in the UK by Athenaeum Press Ltd, Dukesway, Team Valley, Gateshead NE11 0PZ

Dedications

To Jai Maadi for inspiration
and my newly born son, Ishaan Dev
Hitendra Patel

To my wife and son Johann and Julian.
To my mother Louidonne and to the memory
of my father Jean Louis
Jean Joseph

Contents

Contributors

Peter L Acher, Department of Minimally Invasive Surgery and Urology, Whittington Hospital, London, UK

Antonio Alcaraz, Chairman, Department of Urology, Hospital Clinic of Barcelona and Associate Professor of Surgery, University of Barcelona, Spain

Manit Arya, Institute of Urology, University College Hospital, London, UK

Ketan K Badani, Vattikuti Urology Institute, Henry Ford Health Systems, Detroit, Michigan, US

Judd Boczko, Section of Endourology, Laparoscopy, and Robotics, Department of Urology, University of Rochester Medical Center, Rochester, New York, US

Christopher WS Cheng, Department of Urology, Singapore General Hospital, Singapore

Alfred Cutner, Dept of Obstetrics and Gynaecology, University College Hospital, London, UK

Ara Darzi, The Department of Surgery, Anaesthetics and Intensive Care, Imperial College London, UK

Erdal Erturk, Section of Endourology, Laparoscopy, and Robotics, Department of Urology, University of Rochester Medical Center, Rochester, New York, US

Adrian M Harris, Consultant Surgeon, Hinchingbrooke Hospital, Hinchingbrooke Health Care NHS Trust, UK

Ashok K Hemal, Vattikuti Urology Institute, Henry Ford Health Systems, Detroit, Michigan, US

Jean V Joseph, Section of Laparoscopy and Robotics, Department of Urology, University of Rochester Medical Center, Strong Memorial Hospital, Rochester, New York, US

Rohna Kearney, Dept of Obstetrics and Gynaecology, University College Hospital, London, UK

Chryssanthos Kouriefs, Department of Urology, Medway Maritime Hospital, Gillingham, Kent, UK

Tom WJ Lennard, Department of Surgical Sciences, University of Newcastle upon Tyne, UK

Ralph Madeb, Section of Endourology, Laparoscopy, and Robotics, Department of Urology, University of Rochester Medical Center, Rochester, New York, US

Ronald A Miller, Department of Minimally Invasive Surgery and Urology, Whittington Hospital, London, UK

Shikohe Masood, Department of Urology, Medway Maritime Hospital, Gillingham, Kent, UK

Bradley J Nelson, Institute of Robotics and Intelligent Systems, Swiss Federal Institute of Technology (ETH), Zurich, Switzerland

John H Palmer, Department of Urology, Medway Maritime Hospital, Gillingham, Kent, UK

Hitendra Patel, Consultant Laparoscopic Urological Surgeon, Institute of Urology, University College Hospital, London, UK

Edward C Ray, University of Rochester School of Medicine and Dentistry, Department of Surgery, Rochester, New York, US

P S Sains, The Department of Surgery, Anesthetics and Intensive Care, Imperial College London, UK

Luke O Schoeniger, University of Rochester School of Medicine and Dentistry, Department of Surgery, Rochester, New York, US

Iqbal Shergill, Institute of Urology, University College Hospital, London, UK

Kemal B Yesin, Institute of Robotics and Intelligent Systems, Swiss Federal Institute of Technology (ETH), Zurich, Switzerland

Sidney KH Yip, Department of Urology, Singapore General Hospital, Singapore

Anthony Y Young, Department of Minimally Invasive Surgery and Urology, Whittington Hospital, London, UK

Alex Zivanovic, Research Associate, Mechatronics in Medicine Laboratory, Mechanical Engineering Department, Imperial College London, UK

Foreword

Bertrand Guillonneau, MD
Professor of Urology, Head of the Minimally Invasive Surgery section
Department of Urology
Memorial Sloan Kettering Sloan Kettering Cancer Center, New York

Every book of collected essays begins with the visions and predilections of its editor, and this book, too, is a *parti pris* with its enthusiasm for the technological world. This fascination with technical advances should bring, in an obvious way, happiness to those who are likely to benefit from these advances, specifically patients who may live better and longer lives because of this evolution of surgical tools.

This vision of a joyful technology goes back to the 19th century when the emergence of an industrial world made it possible for exploit to follow exploit, on earth, on and under the sea, in the sky, finally reaching into space. The end of the 20th century saw record-breaking achievements in science and the results were spectacular in all fields, medical among others. It is maybe only now that one realizes that this "positivist" attitude has significant costs, financial among others, but in the end, a human cost as well, one which we have hardly begun to take into awareness. A physician often does not want to know of these costs because a doctor's intent to care is laudable by definition and should take precedence over any other consideration, but this does not excuse anyone.

Technology in itself is nothing, and surely not a goal in and of itself, except perhaps in the laboratory where research is concerned. The doctor does not have to take pride in the technology he/she uses, as he/she would not take pride in a scalpel. What has counted and what counts for a surgeon is clinical experience and the mastery of his/her art. In medicine, technology is useful only if it serves the patient and the society in which the patient lives, not the doctor.

Because the use of available techniques for surgical projects goes back far into history, there is a legitimate tendency to think that more technology will add more quality. This is perhaps true in a sense, but it is more likely that one would reach an asymptote, where the technological surplus is more and more expensive for an increasingly reduced medical profit, and where perhaps tomorrow there could be almost no gain of any kind. Perhaps it is already necessary to consider changing the paradigm and to explore how ethical reflections about the patient and the philosophy of the disease, of life and death, will be able to bring more benefit to the sick patient.

And a surgeon is not exempt from thinking.

It is the strength of this book to present an overview of surgical and particularly urological surgery that shows more of the technological, historical, and practical visions of the tools that urology used to become this vast specialty, which came from the simplest medicine, when it was a question of looking at the urine, to the most complex when it became a question of transplanting a kidney. Between these extremes, there is this perspective where the authors invite us to look through the keyhole by adding lenses to see better and by launching micro-robots to be more precise in movement.

Urology is all this, and this is its richness. But it cannot be only that. Our thanks to the authors and the editors for pointing out this naturally exciting reality which inevitably encourages us to question our practice in the world in which we live.

Introduction

Why look through the keyhole?

The introduction of laparoscopy is among the most impressive success stories in the history of medicine. In a relatively short period of time, spanning two to three decades a paradigm shift has occurred where minimally invasive surgery, whether it is endoscopy, laparoscopy, or robot-assisted surgery, has dramatically changed the way surgeons practice medicine. In many disciplines the invasive approaches that were perceived as the norms are quickly being relegated to the past.

The goal of avoiding collateral damage has taken us to a constant renewal process, where procedures are abandoned while they are being replaced by newer, less invasive ones. Surgeons are limiting their contact with the target organ while achieving the same goals. Over the last decade, hand-assisted laparoscopy debuted in many fields. As quickly as it appeared, the challenge to perform these procedures in a completely laparoscopic fashion had begun. While pure laparoscopy is evolving, telesurgery also began its assault on pure laparoscopy, trying to establish its place in the minimally invasive arena, as yet another less invasive approach. As quickly as an invention appears in the surgical arena, its inherent limitations fuel the search for new ones. The field of robotic surgery is gaining momentum, with all its promises, allowing surgeons to perform procedures unparalleled to those previously possible with more invasive techniques. As the use and functionality of robotic surgery evolves, microrobots and eventually nanorobots (some as small as 400 microns in width) will appear in our operating rooms, taking minimally invasive surgery to previously unknown frontiers.

This constant renewal of techniques is coupled with the immense amount of data available to patients in the information age. Patients try to limit the interruption in their lives when they undergo surgical procedures, increasingly seeking procedures that promise a less invasive approach than the ones that may be immediately available to them. The demand for such procedures cannot be overstated. There is an increased demand by patients for treatment options that offer a hastened recovery, decreased post operative pain, and improved cosmesis with similar efficacy to other accepted but rather invasive modalities.

Our aim was to produce an up-to-date book about the most important areas of this new cutting edge technology, with a simplified format allowing non-specialists and specialists to keep abreast of new developments and also refresh their knowledge of historical aspects. We did not wish to make this a reference text, but rather an evolving one.

The evolution of surgical technology will continue, as will the ability of the surgeon to limit the invasiveness of treatment approaches. The news media, the public and surgeons' enthusiasm will continue to fuel this process, and overshadow the lack of long term studies showing safety and efficacy of these newer modalities. Surgeons must be constantly ready to critique procedures both established and new, to determine which ones best meet the goals of minimal invasion to the body, which the patients they serve seek, while delivering an effective treatment. This steady evolution requires a constant retraining and acquisition of new tools which are significant stressors in a cost conscious era. As new promising treatment strategies emerge, the debate will continue on how to best incorporate them in a manner that best benefits the patients and society at large.

Looking through the keyhole offers a glimpse into the vast field of minimally invasive surgery which is developing at breathtaking pace. As surgeons attempt to offer new and better procedures with the help of technology manufacturers, patients will continue to demand better, increasingly critique, and have a voice in the treatment methodology to which they are subjected.

HRH Patel and JV Joseph

CHAPTER 1

Historical development of keyhole surgery

KK Badani, HRH Patel, AK Hemal

The story of modern day laparoscopy began well over a century ago. The pioneers of laparoscopy contributed original ideas and instruments allowing further refinement in optics, safety, and overall acceptance by the medical community eventually culminating into the technology we now use today. This chapter provides a review of important historical events leading up to the current state-of-the-art technology in minimally invasive surgery.

Introduction

Minimally invasive surgery has become a popular alternative to traditional open surgical procedures. Over time laparoscopy has become the standard of care in many common operations, and is readily becoming available for more complex cases in a variety of surgical specialties. If performed safely, endoscopic surgery offers monetary savings in total healthcare as a result of shorter hospital stays and a quicker return to work for most patients. We provide a review of important historical events leading up to the current state-of-the-art technology in minimally invasive surgery.

Historical milestones of endoscopy

The ideas that originally existed and culminated into what we know as laparoscopy today, originated well over a millennium ago. The Arabian physician Abulkasim (936–1013) is cited as the first to inspect the cervix using reflected light. Subsequently, instruments were developed to inspect other body cavities including nasal recesses and urinary bladder (Hemal, 2000). The earliest cystoscope was developed by Philipp Bozzini (*Figure 1.1a*) in 1806 which he termed the 'Lichleiter' (Zucker, 1991; Hemal, 2000) (*Figure 1.1b*). Later, a German scientist,

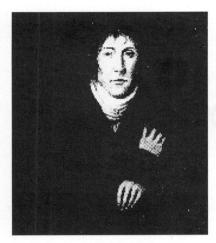

Figure 1.1a: Philipp Bozzini

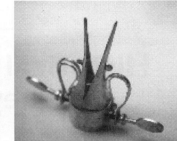

Figure 1.1b: Lichleiter

Maxmillan Nitze developed an instrument in 1877 that more resembles the modern day cystoscope. He incorporated a magnifying optical system with a light source at the tip of the instrument. His light source was an electrically heated platinum wire cooled with a continuous flow of water (Kelly and Burnam, 1914; Mouton *et al*, 1998). This was subsequently modified to an incandescent light source in 1886–1887 due to resultant thermal injury of body tissues (Spaner and Warnock, 1997; Litynski, 1998; Shultheiss *et al*, 1999). It is not surprising, therefore, that cystoscopy preceded all other forms of endoscopy in that the cooling effect of the water flow protected tissues from the thermal injury of the light source.

In 1901, Georg Kelling (Dresden, Germany) (*Figure 1.2*) reported using a cystoscope to inspect the peritoneal cavity of a dog after insufflation with air, a technique he coined 'celioscopy' (Kelling, 1901). Swedish physician Hans Christian Jacobaeus in 1910 performed this procedure in a human (*Figure 1.3*). These early procedures were all diagnostic in nature, as these endoscopes did not allow for adequate exposure and for intervention. It would take another thirty years before pneumoperitoneum was used to facilitate laparoscopy. However, the use of an endoscope through the abdominal wall during this period was subject to a number of complications. The first step in approaching a more safe method of port introduction was modified by Albert Decker (USA) in 1946 where he inserted an endoscope through the cul-de-sac into the abdominal cavity, a procedure he named culdoscopy (Decker, 1946).

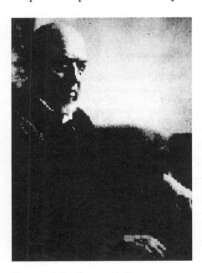

Figure 1.2: Georg Kelling

In 1938, a Hungarian, Janos Veress invented his needle for safe insufflation of air into the abdomen, initially used in the thorax to emulate a pneumothorax. His needle utilized a spring-loaded blunt obturator that self-retracted during penetration of fascial planes, thus protecting the underlying bowel and viscera in the abdomen. Air sufflation at this point was carried

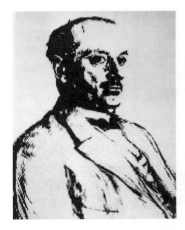

Figure 1.3: HC Jacobaeus

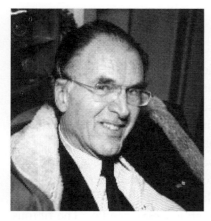

Figure 1.4: Kurt Semm

out with a syringe into the cavity. Raoul Palmer in Paris stressed the importance of monitoring air flow and pressure, however, it was not until twenty years later when Kurt Semm (*Figure 1.4*) in Kiel, Germany, developed a device that automated insufflation while monitoring flow and abdominal pressure (Semm, 1989). With these new developments of safer insufflation and controlling gas flow and pressure during pneumoperitoneum, there was a significant reduction in major complications including bowel perforation and vascular injury (Eisenberg, 1966).

Despite these advances, overall acceptance of these procedures was slow as the quality of images remained quite poor. A striking technological advance, perhaps one of the most significant breakthroughs, came in 1966 when British optical physicist Harold Hopkins developed the rod-lens system. Initial acceptance of his invention was dismal, however, during the course of delivering a lecture in Germany, among his audience members sat Karl Storz, a businessman who owned a firm manufacturing small instruments. His immediate interest in Hopkins' instrument paved the way for the invention that revolutionized endoscopy (Gow, 1998).

The early innovations in the history of endoscopy were advanced by the field of gynecology, led by the German gynecologist Kurt Semm. He is often referred to as the 'father of minimally invasive surgery' as he is credited with making numerous inventions to make laparoscopy a safe procedure. Along with the invention of the automatic insufflation device, he devised the EndoLoop applicator used to prevent loss of pneumoperitoneum during insertion of suture material. Semm then developed the morcellator, an instrument used to remove large portions of tissue. The modern day irrigation-suction apparatus during laparoscopy was made possible by Semm, along with the 'pelvitrainer' used to teach doctors laparoscopic skills (Semm, 1978; Semm, 1979).

Despite the enormous contribution Semm has made to modern day laparoscopy, his ideas were not well received by many surgeons in the 1970s. He performed an entire appendectomy, laparoscopically in 1980 resulting in much animosity and furore (Litynski, 1998). In 1985, Erich Muhe, of Boblingen, Germany, used the technique described by Semm to perform the world's first laparoscopic cholecystectomy. He had a series of ninety-seven cases which he published at the Congress of the German Surgical Society in 1986 (Litynski, 1998). His report did not receive much attention, and was mostly ignored. In the late 1980s, Phillipe Mouret of Lyon, François Dubois, and Jacques of Paris popularized laparoscopic cholecystectomy. In the US, the first laparoscopic cholecystectomy was inspired by a Kurt Semm video of a laparoscopic appendectomy in 1988. McKernan and Save were the two surgeons from Marietta, Georgia, USA who performed this procedure. This was followed by Drs Reddick and Olsen, working in collaboration with McKernan and Save, who published the first clinical report on laparoscopic cholecystectomy (Reddick *et al*, 1989).

Ketan K Badani, Hitendra RH Patel, Ashok K Hemal

Evolution of retroperitoneal laparoscopy

The word laparoscopy, as it is known today, generally implies endoscopic inspection of the peritoneal cavity. Etymologically, *lapara* in Greek means flank, and therefore should denote inspection of the lumbar region. Since this term was initially used for transperitoneal endoscopy, the historical significance remains rather than the literal meaning. Given this history, it seems unavoidable that retroperitoneoscopy would soon follow (Jacobaeus, 1910).

It is well known that early attempts at retroperitoneal laparoscopy were unsuccessful due to uniformly poor results. The inability to create a satisfactory pneumoretroperitoneum was the major obstacle. By mimicking the steps of transperitoneal laparoscopy, these surgeons were unable to create an adequate working space by insufflation through a Veress needle. The fibrous and dense areolar and fatty tissue in the retroperitoneum would not allow adequate insufflation without a disruptive force (Williams *et al*, 1980).

In 1969, Bartel visualized the pelvic retroperitoneum using a mediastinoscope. Similarly, Wittmoser perfomed a retroperitoneal lumbar sympathectomy (Bartel, 1969). Sommerkamp in 1974 performed 'lumboscopy' where he exposed the kidney for renal biopsy (Sommerkamp, 1974). However, access was very limited, visualization remained poor, and the procedures required simplicity. In 1979, John Wickham was the first to perform retroperitoneal laparoscopy using air insufflation and a standard laparoscope. His operation was a ureterolithotomy, and was followed by several others who attempted retroperitoneoscopy (Wickham, 1979). Their efforts were not widely popularized because there still existed an inability to create adequate working space.

More recently, in 1982, Bay-Nielsen and Shultz performed retroperitoneal endoscopic ureterolithotomy using a laryngoscope, and Ralph Clayman *et al* in 1985 performed the operation with an Amplatz sheath (Bay-Nielsen and Schultz, 1982; Clayman *et al*, 1985). Eshgi *et al* in 1985 used a laparoscope to monitor percutaneous transperitoneal removal of a staghorn calculus in a pelvic kidney (Eshghi *et al*, 1985). A historical report in 1991 created worldwide popularity for laparoscopy of retroperitoneal organs when Clayman performed a transperitoneal laparoscopic nephrectomy. Clayman *et al* also performed this operation retroperitoneally, however found this approach unsatisfactory as his exposure with transperitoneal laparoscopy was superior (Clayman *et al*, 1991; Clayman *et al*, 1992). This landmark event led to the modern day urological use of laparoscopy as the standard for minimally invasive surgery of the kidney.

In 1992, Durga Gaur reported an innovative balloon dissection technique of the retroperitoneal space prior to pneumoinsufflation (Gaur *et al*, 1993). The impact of this report was so great that the number of published reports on retroperitoneoscopy more than doubled in a single year. In fact, retroperitoneal laparoscopic nephrectomy has become the procedure of choice for patients with non-functioning kidney and benign symptomatic disease. Ashok Hemal *et al* recently reported on the safety and efficacy of the procedure where he studies a series of 185 retroperitoneal laparoscopic simple nephrectomies with an operative time of 100 minutes, open conversion rate of 10.3% and major complication rate of 3.78% (Hemal *et al*, 2001). As experience has progressed in this area, previously contraindicated complex and trabecular kidneys are safely being removed laparoscopically (Hemal *et al*, 2000).

Evolution of surgical robotics and laparoscopy

'Robot' is derived from a Czech word robota meaning 'forced labor,' a concept that dates back to 3000 BC (Malone, 1996; Shrivastava and Menon, 2002). Automatons, referring to self moving machines, were introduced during the industrial revolution to replace repetitive tasks that were usually performed by human hands. The modern day robot was developed to aid in automation of automobiles. General Motor in 1961 was the first major corporation to use a robot named the Unimate. This machine's function was to 'unload a die-casting machine, quench to hot component, and deliver it to a trim press' (Albus and Engelberger, 1994; Shrivastava and Menon, 2002). This was followed by robotic tasks including lifting heavy machinery, repetitive jobs, and spray-painting car bodies.

The prototype of today's surgical robot was known as 'telcherics' developed at Argonne National Laboratories. This machine used mechanical arms to emulate the movement of a human operator some distance away. This master-slave system formed the ability to take advantage of human cognition and decision-making abilities, and use it towards the robot's fine motor and precision capabilities (Buckingham and Buckingham, 1995). Orthopedics and neurosurgery were the first specialties to take advantage of a robot's fine motor ability. The orthopedic system named RobotDoc (Integrated Surgical Systems, Sacramento, CA) was used for preparing the proximal femur to accept an uncemented total hip prosthesis at a rate ten times faster and 90% more accurate than manual reaming would allow (Paul *et al,* 1992).

During the early 1980s as advancement of optics, video, and instrumentation allowed surgeons to perform more procedures with greater safety, certain laparoscopic operations became the new gold standard including cholecystectomy, Nissen fundoplication, and adrenalectomy. As more complex operations that required fine dissection and reconstruction were attempted, laparoscopists were faced with certain new problems. The most reported problems included a lack of depth perception, limited degrees of freedom (dof), amplification of hand tremor, and counter-intuitive movement of the instruments (Schneeberger and Michler, 2001). As pioneers in minimally invasive surgery were pushing the envelope to advance laparoscopy further, the aforementioned insurmountable difficulties were met with a mix of success and failure. These obstacles were seemingly the driving force in the development of surgical robotics.

Just at a point when enthusiasm for performing all open operations in a laparoscopic fashion was waning, DARPA (Defense Advanced Research Project Administration) was funding tele-surgery research in order to provide surgical care to wounded soldiers in the battlefield from a remote hospital location (Schneeberger and Michler, 2001). In 1993, the Automated Endoscope System for Optimal Positioning (AESOP) from Computer Motion (Goleta, Ca) passed Food and Drug Administration (FDA) approval for clinical use. AESOP uses a six dof arm to mimic the form and function of a human arm to position the endoscope. Later, a voice recognition command system was installed named the HERMES voice control center. Studies performed with this system demonstrated that a robotic device to position the endoscopic camera is more accurate and effective than a human assistant (Kavoussi *et al,* 1995).

The development of a telepresence surgical system for open surgical procedures was led by the Stanford Research Institute (SRI, Stanford, Ca) which subsequently culminated into the establishment of Intuitive Surgical (Mountain View, Ca) in 1995. The initial prototype was built in 1996 and utilized two arms with wristed instruments and six dof. It also included a third camera arm, along with providing stereoscopic vision (Hill *et al*, 1994). This prototype was used for animal trials, and eventually led to a second prototype used to treat humans in Belgium in 1997. An alpha model of the modern daVinci system was developed for cardiac procedures in Paris and Leipzig. Trials for FDA approval were conducted in Mexico City, Mexico, in 1998. By the year 2000, daVinci was approved for laparoscopic use, and in 2001 for thorascopic use. At that time, the daVinci system was used primarily for cardiothoracic procedures, specifically, for in-situ cardiac bypass operations.

Most recently, the thrust of innovation and utilization of the DaVinci system has been in the field of Urology. Robotics has been used in radical prostatectomy, pyeloplasty, radical cystectomy, and female pelvic floor reconstruction to name a few. The primary hindrance of performing such operations in traditional laparoscopic manner is that intra-corporeal suturing in the pelvis using standard laparoscopic instruments has been extremely difficult for most practicing surgeons. This is exemplified by the fact that performance of laparoscopic radical prostatectomy has been performed chiefly in the hands of a few highly skilled surgeons. The articulation afforded by the daVinci system has allowed urologists to perform complex laparoscopic urological operations without the need for 'advanced' laparoscopic skills. Menon *et al* have reported a series of 100 patients undergoing robotic radical prostatectomy using the daVinci system. Their results included a mean operating time of 195 minutes, mean blood loss of 149 mL, and a positive surgical margin rate of 15%. In addition, continence rates were 92% and potency rates of 59% by six months post operatively (Tewari *et al*, 2002; Menon *et al*, 2002; Menon *et al*, 2003).

Although still in its infancy, robotic surgery offers a wide-range of possibilities towards improving current minimally invasive surgical technique, ultimately resulting in improved patient outcomes. Currently at the time of writing this chapter, there are seventy-five daVinci modules in operation in the United States, with another twenty-five in operation outside the U.S.A. With ongoing improvements in both development of hardware and software, physician and patient acceptance, and impact of cost, surgical robotics offers exciting prospects for the future.

Key points for *Chapter 1*

- 936–1013 — Abulkasim first used reflected light to inspect the cervix.
- 1806 — Philipp Bozzini developed the first cystoscope named the 'Lichleiter'.
- 1877 — Maxmillan Nitze refined the cystoscope to include magnified optics and a light source.
- 1901 — Georg Kelling performed 'celioscopy' with air insufflation to inspect the peritoneal cavity of a dog.
- 1910 — Jacobaeus performed the same procedure on a human being.
- 1980 — Kurt Semm performed the first laparoscopic appendectomy.
- 1985 — Muhe performed the first laparoscopic cholecystectomy.
- 1991 — Ralph Clayman performed a transperitoneal laparoscopic nephrectomy.
- 1990s — Defense Advanced Project Research Admininstration funded research for tele-surgery to aid wounded soldiers on the battlefield.
- 2001 — the daVinci surgical system was approved by the FDA and popularized robot-assisted surgery.

References

Albus JS, Engelberger JF (1994) 'Robot.' In: Smith AH (ed) *The Encyclopedia Americana. Danbury*: Grolier Enterprises: 582–85

Bartel M (1969) Die Retroperitoneoskopie. Eine endoscopische Methode zur Inspektion unt bioptischen Untersuchung des retroperitonealen Raumes. *Zentralble Chir* **94**: 377

Bay-Nielsen H, Schultz A (1982) Endoscopic retroperitoneal removal of stones from the upper half of the ureter. *Scand J Urol Nephrol* **16**: 227–28

Buckingham RA, Buckingham RO (1995) Robots in operating theaters. *BMJ* **311**: 1479

Clayman RV, Kavoussi LR *et al* (1992) Laparoscopic nephrectomy: review of the initial 10 cases. *J Endourol* **6**: 127–31

Clayman RV, Kavoussi LR *et al* (1991) Laparoscopic nephrectomy: initial case report. *J Urol* **146**: 278–81

Clayman RV, Preminger GM *et al* (1985) Percutaneous ureterolithotomy. *J Urol* **133**: 671–3

Decker A (1946) Pelvic culdoscopy. In Meigs JV, Sturgis SH, eds. *Progress in Gynecology*. Grune and Stratton, New York

Eisenberg J (1966) On an apparatus for the safe and controllable filling of the abdominal cavity with gas for laparoscopy. *Klin Wochenschr* **44**: 593–4

Eshghi AM, Roth JS *et al* (1985) Percutaneous transperitoneal approach to a pelvic kidney for endourological removal of a staghorn calculus. *J Urol* **134**: 525

Gaur DD, Agarwal DK *et al* (1993) Retroperitoneal laparoscopic nephrectomy: initial case report. *J Urol* **149:** 103–5

Gow JG (1998) Harold Hopkins and optical systems for urology: an appreciation. *Urology* **52:** 152–7

Hemal AK, Gupta NP *et al* (2000) Comparison of retroperitoneoscopic nephrectomy with open surgery for tuberculous nonfunctioning kidneys. *J Urol* **164:** 32–35

Hemal AK, Gupta NP *et al* (2001) Retroperitoneoscopic nephrectomy and nephroureterectomy for benign nonfunctioning kidneys: a single-center experience. *Urology* **57:** 644–49

Hemal AK (2000) *Laparoscopic Urologic Surgery: Retroperitoneal and Transperitoneal.* Churchill Livingstone, New Delhi

Hill J. Green P *et al* (1994) Telepresence surgery demonstration system. Proc. IEEE International Conferences on Robotics Automation, vol 3. San Diego: 2302

Jacobaeus HC (1910) Uber die Maglichkeiten, die Zystoscopie bie Untersuchung seroser Hohlungen anzuwenden. *Munch Med Wochenschr* **57:** 2090–2

Kavoussi LR, Moore RG *et al* (1995) Comparison of robotic versus human laparoscopic camera control. *J Urol* **154:** 2134

Kelling G (1901) Uber Oesophagoskopie, Gastroskopie und Clioskopie. *Munch Med Wochenschr* **49:** 21–4

Kelly HA, Burnam CF (1914) Diseases of the kidneys, ureters and bladder. Appleton, New York

Litynski GS (1998) Kurt Semm and the fight against skepticism: endoscopic hemostasis, laparoscopic appendectomy and Semm's impact on the "laparoscopic revolution." *J Soc Laparoendoscosc Surg* **2:** 309–13

Litynski GS (1998) Endoscopic surgery: the history, the pioneers. *World J Surg* **22:** 745–53

Litynski GS (1998) Erich Muhe and the rejection of laparoscopic cholecystectomy (1985): a surgeon ahead of his time. *JSLS* **2:** 341–6

Malone, Robert (1996) 'Robot.' In: Johnson B (ed.) *Collier's Encyclopedia.* Collier, New York: 115

Menon M, Shrivastava A *et al* (2003) Vattikuti Institute Prostatectomy: a single-team experience of 100 cases. *J Endourol* **17:** 785–90

Menon M, Shrivastava A *et al* (2002) Laparoscopic and robot assisted radical prostatectomy: establishment of a structured program and preliminary analysis of outcomes. *J Urol* **168:** 945–9

Mouton WG, Bessell JR *et al* (1998) Looking back to the advent of modern endoscopy: 150th birthday of Maximilian Nitze. *World J Surg* **22:** 1256–8

Paul HA, Bargar WL *et al* (1992) Development of a surgical robot for cementless total hip replacement. *Clin Orthop* **285:** 57

Reddick EJ, Olson D, *et al* (1989) Laparoscopic laser cholecystectomy. *Laser Med Surg News Adv*: 38–40

Schneeberger WE, Michler RE (2001) An overview of the intuitive system: the surgeon's perspective. *Operative Techniques in Thoracic and Cardiovascular Surgery*: 170

Semm K (1989) History. In Sanfilippo JS, Levine RL (eds) *Operative Gynecologic Endoscopy*. Springer-Verlag, New York

Semm K (1979) New Methods of pelviscopy for myomectomy, ovariectomy, tubectomy and adnectomy. *Endoscopy* **11**: 85–93

Semm K (1978) Tissue-puncher and loop-ligation: new aids for surgical-therapeutic pelviscopy. *Endoscopy* **10**: 119–24

Shrivastava A, Menon M (2002) Surgical Robots: The 'genie' is out. In Hemal AK (ed) *Contemporary trends in laparoscopic urologic surgery*. Churchill Livingstone, New Delhi

Shultheiss D, Machtens SA *et al* (1999) Air cystoscopy: the history of an endoscopic technique from the late 19th century. *BJU Int* **83**: 571–7

Sommerkamp H (1974) Lumboscopie: ein neues diagnostich-therapeutisches Prinzip der urologie. *Acta Urol* **5**: 183

Spaner SJ, Warnock GL (1997) A brief history of endoscopy, laparoscopy, and laparoscopic surgery. *J Laparoendosc Adv Surg Tech A* **7**: 369–73

Tewari A, Peabody J *et al* (2002) Technique of da Vinci robot-assisted anatomic radical prostatectomy. *Urology* **60**: 569–72

Wickham JEA (ed) (1979) The surgical treatment of renal lithiasis. In: Urinary calculus disease. Churchill Livingstone, New York: 145–98

Williams PL, Warwick R (1980) Myology. In: Williams and Warwick. *Gray's anatomy*, 36th ed Churchill Livingstone, Edinburgh: 506–93

Zucker KA, Bailey RW *et al* (1991) *Surgical Laparoscopy*. Quality Medical Pub, St. Louis

UNIVERSITIES AT MEDWAY LIBRARY

CHAPTER 2

Diagnostic laparoscopic general surgery

AM Harris, HRH Patel, TWJ Lennard

Laparoscopy as a diagnostic tool maybe used in an emergency or an elective setting. In the former it is most commonly used with penetrating trauma and for suspected appendicitis. Electively a diagnostic laparoscopy may be performed on patients with chronic undiagnosed abdominal pain or staging modalities in upper gastro intestinal and hepatobiliary cancers. We review diagnostic laparoscopy and the potential applications.

Introduction

Laparoscopy has moved from the research arena to established procedure but there remains a wide spectrum of acceptance and usage both in terms of technological limitations and philosophical approach. While some procedures have now become the 'gold standard' of treatment, for example cholecystectomy, at the other end of the spectrum there is still debate over the use of laparoscopy in cancer surgery. The whole approach to laparoscopic surgery now benefits from the establishment of standardized training protocols and significant technological input from the manufacturing companies together with surgeons at the forefront of the pioneering work, who are continually looking for ways to improve efficiency and safety. There is no doubt that major advancements have been made in the last ten years principally because of technological development creating instrumentation which maintains high quality and strength without compromising functionality. This chapter provides an overview of diagnostic laparoscopy.

The use of laparoscopy as a diagnostic tool may be used either in the emergency or the elective setting (Riemann, 2003). In the former it is most commonly used with penetrating trauma and for suspected appendicitis particularly in young females where other pathology may be responsible for the symptoms. Electively a diagnostic laparoscopy (DL) may be performed on patients with chronic undiagnosed abdominal pain when either adhesions or occult inflammation may be suspected. It is also used as one of the staging modalities in upper gastro intestinal and hepatobiliary cancers.

AM Harris, HRH Patel, TWJ Lennard

Emergency laparoscopy

Trauma

The use of DL in the management of penetrating abdominal trauma was first considered in the late 1970s (Simon *et al*, 2002). In a haemodynamically stable patient with an abdominal wall stab wound, the likelihood of peritoneal penetration is sometimes equivocal on superficial wound exploration, and it was therefore postulated that laparoscopy would confirm the extent of injury and thus potentially reduce the number of negative laparotomies. However this approach was not widely adopted until relatively recently, and the review by the teams with the earliest experience appeared to demonstrate a reduction in unnecessary laparotomy with the end benefit of laparoscopic repair of visceral or diaphragmatic injury. It has been recommended that this should be used as a diagnostic tool in the stable patient, in a unit with appropriate training and equipment with the technique of systematic laparoscopic abdominal exploration (Gorecki *et al*, 2002).

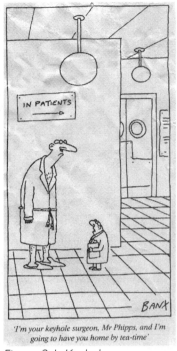

'I'm your keyhole surgeon, Mr Phipps, and I'm going to have you home by tea-time'

Figure 2.1: Keyhole surgeon

There is considerable debate in the medical press at the present time over the use of DL in the trauma patient. A differentiation must be made between blunt and penetrating abdominal trauma. Blunt trauma typically involves a greater degree of kinetic energy to a larger area of the body. These injuries are usually severe leading to haemodynamic instability, therefore requiring early laparotomy (Leppaniemi and Elliott, 1996). Penetrating trauma may be confined to a smaller area of the abdominal cavity, and is more likely to cause injuries that would be accessible to the laparoscope. However some centres have expressed concern over the possibility of occult injuries either to the diaphragm or hollow viscus, leading to a false negative result at laparoscopic exploration. In the medical literature opinion remains divided. A randomized trial from Finland incorporated a DL into the routine diagnostic work-up of patients with abdominal stab wounds comparing the overall results between exploratory laparotomy and DL. They also looked at patients with equivocal peritoneal violation on local wound exploration who were then randomised either to DL or expectant non-operative management. They found that in patients with demonstrated peritoneal violation there was no difference between the two groups, and in those with equivocal peritoneal penetration more minor organ injuries were detected laparoscopically but this was associated with increased hospital stay and costs. They concluded that this approach cannot be recommended as a routine diagnostic tool in antero-lateral abdominal and thoraco-abdominal stab wounds. However the same group also looked at the incidence of missed occult diaphragmatic injuries in stable patients, who may subsequently develop late herniation and visceral strangulation. After excluding patients with other injuries requiring surgical repair, during which these injuries would be diagnosed and treated, they found an overall risk of 7% occult diaphragmatic injury, and recommend consideration of DL or thoracoscopy particularly in left sided stab wounds (Leppaniemi and Haapiainen, 2003).

In summary, whilst the literature is divided it would appear that in centers with the expertise and equipment, it would be appropriate to perform a DL on stable patients with a view to obtaining an accurate diagnosis of internal injury, avoidance of unnecessary laparotomy and repair of visceral or diaphragmatic injuries when found (Zantut *et al*, 1997; Chol and Lim, 2003). Clearly there is potential for catastrophic injury with penetrating wounds and the overall philosophy of care for these patients must involve regular monitoring of haemodynamic parameters and regular review of clinical signs and symptoms. If there is any doubt about intra-abdominal injury then an open laparotomy is mandatory.

Appendicitis

The use of laparoscopy in appendicitis has been extensively reported in the medical literature. As laparoscopic techniques have become more available and technological advances have improved instrumentation, there has been an increase in use of this mode of investigation and treatment for appendicitis. An objective comparison between the laparoscopic or the open approach needs to discern a real benefit to the patient, and typically parameters of hospital stay, post-operative pain, and interval to resuming normal activities have been assessed. The literature is equivocal with some reports finding no difference between the two approaches, concluding that the use of laparoscopic appendectomy should be confined to those with specific training and appropriate equipment, but not universally recommended. Other groups have found a small but significant decrease in analgesia requirements and also shorter time to resume normal activities (Hellberg *et al*, 1999). The length of hospital stay is more equivocal with a possible reduction of one day (Marzouk *et al*, 2003; Guller *et al*, 2004). The routine use of the laparoscopic approach is not yet recommended as a gold standard, but this is probably due to the availability of equipment and training (Noble *et al*, 2003) and there is little doubt that in time it will become the procedure of choice. There is however current consensus of benefit in young women of child-bearing age who have signs and symptoms suggestive of appendicitis but clinical examination is more equivocal. Initial laparoscopy in these cases will not only confirm or refute a diagnosis of appendicitis, but also enable adequate visualization of the pelvic organs and in particular the left ovary and fallopian tube, which are often inaccessible with the open approach. Where pelvic pathology is found, appropriate procedures can be undertaken laparoscopically including biopsy or aspiration of cysts, tubal surgery, or indeed no procedure at all (van Dalen *et al*, 2003). Whether or not to continue with appendicectomy if the appendix is found to be normal is debated among experts, but on balance it would be reasonable to remove the appendix firstly because in the absence of any other defined pathology the appendix is accessible and its removal will prevent the possibility of subsequent admissions with similar symptoms in the future. Secondly it is recognized that appendicitis can present without any obvious inflammation on visual inspection, if caught early enough. Histology in these cases may show high aggregation of lymphocytes sub mucosally confirming appendicitis in an otherwise healthy looking appendix (Navez and Therasse, 2003). Finally, it has been suggested that the presentation of an appendix mass is a contraindication to the laparoscopic approach. This view has been recently challenged with one small study demonstrating this to be a feasible and safe procedure with no difference in outcome between mass- and non-mass appendicectomies, and the added advantage of avoidance of a second hospital admission (Senapathi *et al*, 2003).

AM Harris, HRH Patel, TWJ Lennard

Elective laparoscopy

Staging laparoscopy

This modality is used particularly in upper gastro intestinal and hepatobiliary cancers when patients are being staged prior to decisions concerning their management. Gastric and junctional tumours may extend to the serosa with subsequent peritoneal seeding of tumour cells and development of ascites. In such cases surgical treatment is contraindicated and where this is suspected a staging laparoscopy is performed. This will reveal small hepatic metastases which may have been missed by CT scan, and will also allow aspiration cytology and biopsy of suspicious peritoneal lesions. If any of these are positive then the patient is saved from a major surgical procedure with its accompanying risk of mortality and morbidity and will be more appropriately managed with palliative treatment such as chemotherapy, allowing a better quality of life in the terminal phase of the disease.

Chronic abdominal pain

A diagnostic laparoscopy may also be considered for patients with chronic undiagnosed abdominal pain in whom no pathology has been found after extensive investigation. Occasionally this will reveal an occult lesion or adhesions which may be either congenital or secondary to previous surgery, and these may be dealt with laparoscopically leading to resolution of symptoms (Kavic, 2002). Alternately a negative laparoscopy would provide reassurance of a lack of obvious pathology and the patient may then be treated for a functional disorder with more confidence.

Key points for *Chapter 2*

- Diagnostic laparoscopy is useful in penetrating trauma to avoid unnecessary laparotomy in the stable patient, but occult injuries may be missed. It may also be helpful in the management of chronic abdominal pain.

- Laparoscopic appendectomy is recommended in younger females or when the diagnosis is in doubt, but the technique is mainly limited to specialist centres at present.

- Staging laparoscopy is utilized in upper gastrointestinal and hepatobiliary cancer to identify patients with inoperable disease who will avoid radical surgery and proceed to palliative treatment.

References

Chol YB and KS Lim (2003) Therapeutic laparoscopy for abdominal trauma. *Surg Endosc* **17(3):** 421–7

Gorecki PJ *et al* (2002) Diagnostic and therapeutic laparoscopy for trauma: a technique of safe and systematic exploration. *Surg Laparosc Endosc Percutan Tech* **12(3):** 195–8

Guller U *et al* (2004) Laparoscopic versus open appendectomy: outcomes comparison based on a large administrative database. *Ann Surg* **239(1):** 43–52

Hellberg A *et al* (1999) Prospective randomized multicentre study of laparoscopic versus open appendicectomy. *Br J Surg* **86(1):** 48–53

Kavic SM (2002) Adhesions and adhesiolysis: the role of laparoscopy. *Jsls* **6(2):** 99–109

Leppaniemi A and Haapiainen R (2003) Occult diaphragmatic injuries caused by stab wounds. *J Trauma* **55(4):** 646–50

Leppaniemi AK and DC Elliott (1996) The role of laparoscopy in blunt abdominal trauma. *Ann Med* **28(6):** 483–9

Marzouk M *et al* (2003) Laparoscopic versus open appendectomy: a prospective comparative study of 227 patients. *Surg Endosc* **17(5):** 721–4

Navez B and A Therasse (2003) Should every patient undergoing laparoscopy for clinical diagnosis of appendicitis have an appendicectomy? *Acta Chir Belg* **103(1):** 87–9

Noble H, P Gallagher *et al* (2003) Who is doing laparoscopic appendicectomies and who taught them? *Ann R Coll Surg Engl* **85(5):** 331–3

Riemann JF, Agresta F *et al* (2000) Emergency laparoscopy: a community hospital experience. *Surg Endosc* **14(5):** 484-7

Simon RJ, Rabin J *et al* (2002) Impact of increased use of laparoscopy on negative laparotomy rates after penetrating trauma. *J Trauma* **53(2):** 297–302; discussion 302

Senapathi PS, D Bhattacharya *et al* (2002) Early laparoscopic appendectomy for appendicular mass. *Surg Endosc* **16(12):** 1783–5

van Dalen R, Bagshaw PF *et al* (2003) The utility of laparoscopy in the diagnosis of acute appendicitis in women of reproductive age. *Surg Endosc* **17(8):** 1311–3

Zantut LF *et al* (1997) Diagnostic and therapeutic laparoscopy for penetrating abdominal trauma: a multicenter experience. *J Trauma* **42(5):** 825–9; discussion 829–31

CHAPTER 3

Therapeutic laparoscopic general surgery

AM Harris, HRH Patel, TWJ Lennard

Laparoscopy as a therapeutic tool is gaining popularity. The commonest areas of use include biliary, anti-reflux, morbid obesity, colorectal, and endocrine surgery. The important considerations in the application of laparoscopy as a therapeutic tool are reviewed.

Introduction

The explosion in interest and application of laparoscopic surgery took place in the late 1980s and it was in the field of hepatobiliary surgery, particularly the surgery for gallstones that the early expansion of this minimally invasive technology took place. The pioneers of laparoscopic biliary surgery were a driving force for the application of this novel way of operative intervention, however the technological development enabling good quality images to be transmitted from the laparoscope to a screen, coupled with instrumentation, played a major part.

Biliary surgery

The early pioneers of laparoscopic cholecystectomy made a point of recommending that the indications for surgery and the basic steps in the operation should remain identical to those for the open operation. Thus the indications for referral for gall bladder laparoscopic surgery remain, in the vast majority of cases, the treatment of symptomatic gallstones. There were concerns that once the technology was introduced and the efficacy of the operation proven, that surgeons would be tempted to operate on cases via the laparoscopic route that they wouldn't have recommended open surgery for, but this has not been the case. All patients with symptomatic gallstones should therefore be considered for laparoscopic cholecystectomy and there will only be a few instances where this will not be possible or advisable (Downs *et al*, 1996). This will include any concerns

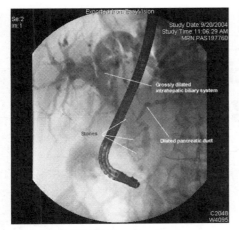

Figure 3.1: ERCP Showing large gallstones impacted in the CBD which could not be removed endoscopically. Distal impaction is causing distension of the pancreatic duct. These stones were successfully removed at laparoscopic exploration of CBD

that the gall bladder may be the seat of malignant disease. Gall bladder carcinoma is a rare disease. It is nearly always associated with gallstones and is not commonly diagnosed preoperatively. Nevertheless in those few cases where laparoscopic surgery has been done for cases where there has been a coexistent gall bladder carcinoma concerns have been raised about possible seeding in port sites and adequacy of tumour clearance.

Previous upper abdominal surgery and even known common bile duct stones may be relative contraindications to laparoscopic surgery but a trial of dissection will often prove that the laparoscopic route is possible. If at all possible known common bile duct stones should be removed prior to the laparoscopic removal of the gall bladder using endoscopic retrograde cholangiopancreatography (ERCP) together with sphincterotomy and stone retrieval. Where this is not possible through the lower bile duct preoperatively it is now possible to explore the common bile duct laparoscopically and remove stones from the common duct in the same way as at open operation (*Figures 3.1 and 3.2*).

Patients with known portal hypertension can be operated on safely laparoscopically for removal of the gall bladder and the same care must be taken with friable varices as would be the case at open surgery. Patients undergoing chronic ambulatory peritoneal dialysis and with ventriculoperitoneal shunts can also undergo laparoscopic removal of the gall bladder.

In discussing the operation with the patient, clearly the clinician must cover the possibility of the need to convert to an open operation. Within the UK approximately 9% of patients overall will need conversion to an open procedure although in specialist centres this falls to <5%. Individual surgeons should know their own conversion rate and explain this to the patient. Previous surgery in the right upper quadrant, morbid obesity, repeated episodes of cholecystitis, suspicion of empyema and the presence of common bile duct stones will all make conversion more likely. Neither the surgeon nor the patient should be concerned if conversion has to happen and it should not be considered a failure but simply a prudent step that the operator should have no hesitation in taking if at any time during the laparoscopic procedure progress is not safe and satisfactory. Day case laparoscopic cholecystectomy is becoming standard policy in many units and the routine use of postoperative drains is not commonly practised, thereby allowing early discharge. Pre- or perioperatively the patient should be given antibiotics as prophylaxis against infection recognising that bile is commonly colonized by organisms such as Escherichia coli, *streptococcus faecalis* and anaerobes.

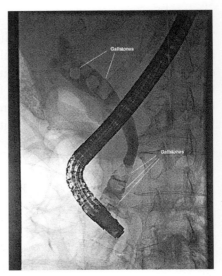

Figure 3.2: ERCP showing large impacted gallstones in both the Common Hepatic Duct and the Common Bile Duct which could not be removed endoscopically. These stones were successfuly removed at laparoscopic exploration of CBD

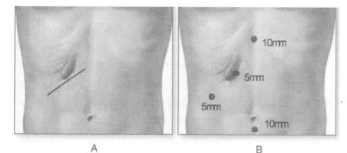

A   B

Figure 3.3: Surgical approach to cholecystectomy.
(A) Kocher's incision for open surgery; (B) Port sites for
laparoscopic access. The camera is usually placed into the
umbilical port

The question of laparoscopic perioperative cholangiography is controversial. The majority of surgeons in the UK do not perform perioperative cholangiograms routinely but there are those who do in the knowledge that silent common bile duct stones occur in a small proportion of patients. The cholangiogram can be used to confirm anatomy and on occasions salvage a situation which might otherwise require conversion if structures are indistinct (Berci *et al*, 1991; Flum *et al*, 2003).

The careful placement of ports to perform the operation is essential (*Figure 3.3*). The first port site traditionally developed is the periumbilical one. Most operators now will cut down under direct vision into the peritoneal cavity rather than using a Veress needle. This allows safe placement of a 10mm diameter blunt port into the abdomen and the creation of a pneumoperitoneum. Carbon dioxide is used to establish the pneumoperitoneum and an intra-abdominal pressure of around 12mm of mercury would normally be sufficient to create enough space for the rest of the operation to proceed. Once the first port site has been inserted and the pneumoperitoneum established a further upper port of 10mm diameter can be inserted under direct vision angulating the port through the abdominal wall to minimize the risk of port site hernia and aiming to enter the peritoneal cavity just to the right of the falciform ligament. Two lateral 5mm ports are then inserted in the right subcostal position to allow most laterally a retractor for the gall bladder fundus and more medially the left hand instrument, commonly an atraumatic grasper. Through the upper 10mm port site the main operating instruments will be placed and the instruments used for dissection will include diathermy scissors, blunt dissection with pledgets and a suction-irrigation device. The basic principles of the operation involve a careful display of the anatomy, and in particular Calot's triangle. Retraction of the gall bladder fundus by the most lateral grasper into the space created by the pneumoperitoneum is required, and it may on occasion be necessary to take down adhesions before this can be achieved. Using a combination of sharp, diathermy and blunt dissection the gall bladder fundus is traced down to the cystic duct/common bile duct junction and at this point, if required, a perioperative cholangiogram can be performed. A variety of instruments exist to facilitate perioperative cholangiography and a further technique of value is the simple placement of an 18-gauge intravenous long line through the abdominal wall acting as a fifth port and leaving both hands and operating ports free for the manipulation of the catheter into the common bile duct. Once the cholangiogram has been completed the cystic duct is clipped using reusable or disposable clip applicators. It can then be divided along with the cystic artery once that has also been clipped. Traction on Hartmanns pouch then displays the anatomy and allows the gall bladder to be dissected off the liver bed using hook diathermy dissection. The right upper quadrant can be washed and sucked out using a suction irrigation system if necessary. Drains can be placed through one of the most lateral port sites if required and the gall bladder removed through either of the 10mm port sites. To facilitate removal of the gall bladder it is commonly placed inside a retrieval bag. The pneumoperitoneum is then released, port sites removed and the 10mm port sites closed with an absorbable suture to the aponeurosis and subcuticular sutures to the skin. The 5mm port sites can be closed with Steri-strips alone. All port sites are infiltrated with local anesthetic at the end of the procedure.

Complications from laparoscopic cholecystectomy are uncommon. It is exceptionally unusual to see subphrenic abscess, though bile leaks do occur and can be managed conservatively by percutaneous drainage or sometimes ERCP and stent placement. Hemorrhage is uncommon and may require open operation to control it. Damage to the bile duct can occur if structures have been misidentified, ligaclips misplaced or diathermy used close to the common bile duct. Suspected bile duct damage should be repaired at the time if it is recognised, and if not, should be referred into a specialist centre for investigation and appropriate management once it is identified (Dunn *et al*, 1994). Wound problems are rare with laparoscopic cholecystectomy but port site herniation can occur if the deep layers have not been closed appropriately.

Upper gastrointestinal surgery

The use of laparoscopy in upper gastrointestinal surgery has increased significantly over the past decade. Initially this was confined to benign procedures such as repair of hiatus hernia and anti-reflux surgery, and more latterly has been extended to cancer surgery.

Anti-reflux surgery

The first Laparoscopic Nissen Fundoplication for severe gastro-oesophageal reflux disease (GORD) was performed in 1992 and since then has gained a wide acceptance in specialist centers with overall results approaching 90% success. Patients must have appropriate counselling from a Specialist Laparoscopic Surgeon with regard to the nature and complications of the treatment. Typically they will present with an appropriate history of reflux disease, and a subsequent endoscopy will confirm varying degrees of erosive esophagitis or indeed the presence of Barrett's esophagus. Esophageal pH and manometry studies are essential firstly to exclude esophageal dysmotility as a potential cause of reflux symptoms and secondly to confirm and quantify the reflux symptoms. There is usually (but not always) a hiatus hernia involved and the procedure, as in open surgery, involves adequate dissection of the hiatus, crural repair, and reconstruction of an anti-reflux valve which may either be a full 360° wrap (true Nissen Fundoplication – *Figure 3.4*) or a variety on this technique of either posterior (Toupet) or anterior (Watson) 180° repair.

There has been debate over the need to divide the short gastric arteries (SGA) in order to adequately mobilize the fundus (Richardson and Hunter, 1999). A prospective study from Adelaide found no benefit at five-year follow-up, and in fact quoted a significant increase in wind-related problems with division of SGA (Chrysos *et al*, 2001; O'Boyle *et al*, 2002). Long term success of this operation is 90–95% (Granderath *et al*, 2002) and the patient must clearly understand the risk of failure, in which case further surgery may be required. Side-effects include gas bloat syndrome where the patient may experience acute gastric dilatation in the early postoperative phase and for this reason they are advised to stick to fluid and soft diet only with the avoidance of alcohol and fizzy drinks. A further postoperative complication is dysphagia which in the majority of cases

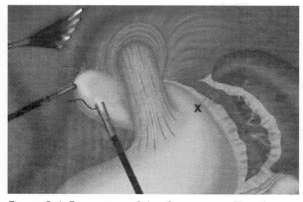

Figure 3.4: Formation of the floppy wrap. The Crura have been tightened and the short gastric arteries divided to mobilize the fundus, which has been taken behind the oesophagus. It will be sutured to the anterior fundal wall (x)

settles within a few days or weeks without the requirement of further treatment. Where dysphagia persists a simple endoscopy may relieve symptoms, but dilatation may also be required. If the patient remains symptomatic, or suddenly becomes dysphagic after vomiting, re-operation is indicated as this suggests possible slippage of the wrap. Surgery may involve taking down the wrap with subsequent re-do fundoplication or a refinement to the partial wrap. In exceptional cases the wrap may need to be fully dismantled. In this instance it is accepted that the patient will need to return to anti-reflux medication, but surprisingly in some cases they remain relatively asymptomatic and no further treatment is required.

Morbid obesity

A number of surgical options exist for the treatment of morbid obesity. These include gastric banding and gastric diversion with a variety of methods of reconstruction. However, in addition to the usual risks associated with any surgical procedure there are particular risks to the patient because of their size, and it is only undertaken in specialist centres. All of the techniques employed in open surgery are eminently suitable for the laparoscopic approach and this has now become a standard treatment in those laparoscopic centres with an interest in bariatric surgery (Herron, 2004).

Obesity is defined as a BMI greater than thirty, with morbid obesity BMI greater than forty and super-obesity BMI greater than fifty. Surgery is usually undertaken on patients in the age range 18–60, who have undergone at least one year of dietary failure and have been clinically obese for five years or more. They should have minimal risks with regard to co-morbidity and it is also recommended that they are assessed by a Psychiatrist and that there should be no history of drug addiction. They will undergo an intensive preoperative work-up including cardiopulmonary, endocrine, gastrointestinal and psychological investigation. The treatment is considered effective if the patient loses greater than 50% of their excess weight with few complications.

Gastric banding involves the placement of a prosthetic band around the upper part of the stomach, which creates a small upper chamber of the stomach leading to early satiety when eating (Ren *et al*, 2004). A vertical banded gastroplasty involves a similar type of banding with the addition of vertical stapling of the fundus to exclude the upper part of the stomach. Gastric diversion is a method of reducing the capacity of the stomach followed by Roux-en-Y reconstruction and there are a variety of anastomotic modifications, including biliopancreatic bypass with a duodenal switch (Lee *et al*, 2004; Weiner *et al*, 2004). Complications of these procedures include those common to any laparoscopic procedure including intraoperative visceral injury and hemorrhage.

They can develop early or late postoperative complications. The early group includes immediate dysphagia and slipped band. In the late postoperative group some patients suffer with pouch formation where the gastric reservoir proximal to the band becomes distended into a large pouch which then fails to empty completely. This is usually due to the ingestion of large meals despite advice to the contrary. Other late complications include perforation, gastric erosion and mechanical problems with the catheter (Smith *et al*, 2004, Chevallier *et al*, 2004). With regard to outcomes of this type of surgery, success has been somewhat arbitrarily defined as a sustained loss of at least 50% of initial excess weight (IEWL). The results in most series are favourable with IEWL rates reported between 45 and 75% (O'Brien and Dixon, 2003; Moose *et al*, 2003) but this will depend on length of follow-up. A more significant outcome of this type of surgery is the effect on comorbidity associated with obesity. Conditions that have been improved or cured include type II diabetes, hypertension, osteoarthritis, hyperlipidaemia, obstructive sleep apnoea, urinary stress incontinence and GORD. Risk of MI and CVA is reduced. Furthermore there is evidence from the pre-laparoscopic era that the increased mortality associated with morbid obesity reverts to a normal risk after successful bariatric surgery (Benotti *et al*, 1989). Success will mainly be influenced by surgical experience, patient selection and in particular patient motivation and it must be stressed that psychological and dietary assessment is mandatory in these patients prior to consideration for an operation.

Surgery for cancer

At the present time the primary treatment for both gastric and esophageal carcinoma with curative intent remains surgical excision. There is currently a significant amount of research being carried out into the role of chemotherapy and radiotherapy with early trials suggesting small but definite benefits in a selective group of patients. The laparoscopic approach has not yet been widely adopted, currently being carried out in only a few specialist centres within defined research protocols (Nguyen *et al*, 2001; Luketich *et al*, 2003). Total gastrectomy and sub-total esophagectomy are major surgical undertakings, technically demanding and carrying considerable risk of morbidity and mortality. The possibility of a laparoscopic approach is therefore viewed with a degree of surgical scepticism in some centres particularly over the success rate with regard to negative resection margins and lymphadenectomy. However a number of series appear to demonstrate good early results, although the follow up is understandably short (Luketich *et al*, 2003; Weber *et al*, 2003; Shimizu *et al*, 2003). Overall it is probably fair to say that the long term results from the few centers undertaking this type of laparoscopic surgery will be watched closely and with great interest by the upper gastrointestinal surgical community, and as experience and technology progress it will probably gain greater acceptance as a treatment option. The advantages to the patient obviously include those of any laparoscopic procedure with reduced postoperative pain, early mobilization and discharge from hospital and the concomitant reduction in risk of systemic complications.

The typical approach for an esophagectomy would include standard laparoscopic set up and full mobilization of the stomach and esophagus via the diaphragmatic hiatus. This dissection can then be carried out further up into the chest. The operator gains access to the proximal esophagus via a neck incision; the stomach is pulled up into the chest, the tumor resected and an extracorporeal anastomosis performed. Alternatively, thoracoscopic access may be used to continue the esophageal dissection and perform the anastomosis (Nguyen *et al*, 2003). Gastrectomy is performed with the same principals as the open procedure, and recently has been described with the addition of a plastic cushion device to allow the surgeons hand access to the abdominal compartment without loss of pneumoperitoneum (Glasgow and Swantstrom, 2001). This has been called Hand-Assisted Laparoscopic Surgery (HALS) and is described in more detail below.

Colorectal surgery

Most colorectal procedures have been attempted laparoscopically, but once again this is usually within the province of a specialist or research unit. However, acceptance of the laparoscopic approach is increasing and a number of centres now have considerable series of patients undergoing surgery for both benign and malignant conditions (Chung *et al*, 2003). Benign laparoscopic colorectal surgery is rapidly gaining acceptance, eg. colectomy for diverticular disease (Guller *et al*, 2003), but there remains considerable debate in the literature over the laparoscopic approach to cancer surgery. Concerns include the adequacy of resection and port site recurrences. Furthermore, the laparoscopic approach usually, but not invariably, involves a longer operating time although this would be expected to reduce with increasing experience and expertise. Nevertheless current opinion in the medical literature is divided. A large multi-centered trial from America comparing laparoscopically-assisted colectomy with the open approach did find modest benefits with the laparoscopic operation, particularly with less analgesic requirement and shorter postoperative stay in hospital. However the conclusion was of a modest benefit which did not justify the routine use of laparoscopic surgery for these patients (Weeks *et al*, 2002). Conversely Lacy et al found an improved five-year survival despite a high recurrence rate at 27%. They concluded that the laparoscopic approach was as good as open surgery and should be offered to patients (Lacy *et al*, 2002). Both of these studies have flaws which will raise questions over their conclusions. It remains a hotly debated topic and a review of the available published data needs to be undertaken with caution. Recent studies report favourable outcomes with laparoscopic surgery (Yamamoto *et al*, 2002; Patankar *et al*, 2003; Tsang *et al*, 2003), even in the elderly population (Weber, 2003), but longer postoperative follow up will be required before the evidence is sufficient for a definitive conclusion (Anthuber *et al*, 2003).

Endocrine surgery

Laparoscopic surgery for the adrenal gland, the spleen and the kidney has expanded significantly in the last five years. Disorders of these glands are uncommon so the overall experience in any given centre is more limited compared to gall bladder surgery and the management of more common diseases. Nevertheless the indications for adrenal laparoscopic surgery encompass virtually all diseases of the adrenal gland with the possible exception of malignant tumours. There are early concerns that the management of adrenal malignant tumours laparoscopically may lead to increased rates of tumour bed recurrence and therefore most endocrine laparoscopic surgeons would avoid operating on a known or suspected adrenal carcinoma. Benign adenomas of the adrenal that produce Cushing syndrome aldosterone-secreting tumours (Conn's syndrome) and phaeochromocytomas are all eminently treatable by laparoscopic adrenalectomy (Gagner *et al*, 1992). Large adrenal tumours up to 15cm in size can be removed laparoscopically and bilateral adrenal lesions can also be removed in a synchronous operation (Henry *et al*, 2002). For functioning adrenal masses it is essential where possible to have control of the endocrine output of the glands prior to surgical removal (Patel *et al*, 2001). This is particularly important in relation to phaeochromocytoma. Any concern that the contralateral gland if this is to be left in place is functioning or capable of functioning should be addressed to avoid postoperative Addisonian crisis. Previous surgery in or around the area of the adrenal gland is not normally a major problem as adhesions can be taken down and the adrenal gland by virtue of its retroperitoneal position will commonly be unaffected by peritoneal cavity adhesions. A trans-peritoneal approach is most commonly utilized though pure retroperitoneal tunnelling approaches have been described and have a role. In the trans-peritoneal operation the patient will be positioned typically on their side with a break in the table to open the space between the costal margin and the anterior superior iliac spine. The first port site on the left side to be inserted will be inserted under direct vision by cutting down into the peritoneal cavity just below the costal margin. Care should be taken in the placement of this port to avoid damage to the splenic flexure of the colon and once the port has been inserted under direct vision a pneumoperitoneum can be established. Two further ports will then typically be required, one halfway between the umbilicus and the costal margin for the camera and another medially in the subcostal margin for the left handed instrument to be placed. Once all instruments are in the abdomen it may be necessary to take down the splenic flexure of the colon to allow access to the left subphrenic space. The lienorenal ligament must be divided and either diathermy or high frequency ultrasonic dissectors can be used to do this. This allows the spleen to be retracted medially and open up the space above the kidney where the adrenal gland will be found. Identifying the gland can be difficult if it is small and in an obese (eg. Cushingoid) patient. Landmarks to finding the gland include the upper pole of the kidney and the renal vein. Care must be taken not to damage the pancreas or the spleen as dissection proceeds. The adrenal and its associated pathology will be friable and care should be taken not to fragment it as the tissues around the gland are cleared. Numerous feeding vessels particularly evident in phaeochromocytoma will need to be controlled using the harmonic scalpel or diathermy and where appropriate using ligaclips. The adrenal vein on the left side drains into the renal vein and this should be formally identified and secured with clips. Once mobilised the adrenal gland can be placed inside a retrieval bag and removed through one of the port sites. It is commonly not necessary to leave a drain down to the bed of dissection but one can be placed through one of the port sites if required. Once the pneumoperitoneum has been released the 10mm port sites can be closed with an absorbable suture to the external muscle aponeurosis and with Steri-strips or subcutaneous stitches to the skin. On the right side the patient will be lying right side up again with a table break. The first port site should be placed in the subcostal position, care being taken to avoid any damage to a low-lying liver. If done under direct vision this is not difficult and the pneumoperitoneum can be easily established once the port is in place. A further two ports will be needed and possibly a third if a liver retractor is required. These will be placed for the camera halfway between the umbilicus and the costal margin and for the operating port sites more laterally in a subcostal position. Identification of the inferior vena cava and retraction of the right lobe of the liver is required. The peritoneum overlying the posterior abdominal wall and the adrenal gland can be divided using the harmonic scalpel and the adrenal gland will commonly be seen easily lying close to inferior vena cava and the hilum of the liver. Mobilization of the gland can proceed from the lower pole upwards running alongside the inferior vena cava securing any small draining vessels with ligaclips or the harmonic scalpel. Care should be taken in identifying and formally securing the adrenal vein which on the right side drains directly into the vena cava. This should be secured with ligaclips. Once mobilization of the glands has been completed it can be placed into a retrieval bag and removed. The port sites are infiltrated with local anesthetic and closed in a similar fashion to the left side.

Bilateral laparoscopic adrenalectomy can be easily performed by simply turning the patient from side to side once the first gland has been removed.

Laparoscopic splenectomy can be performed as can removal of the rare cysts of the spleen with relative ease. Indications include hereditary spherocytosis, idiopathic thrombocytopaenia and hypersplenism. Massively enlarged spleens are not easily removed laparoscopically but moderately enlarged and normal sized spleens are relatively easily approached through similar placement of ports for a left adrenal gland. Again the lienorenal ligament is mobilized. Movement of the table may be required to optimize the use of gravity in splenectomy and allowing the short gastric vessels to be secured between ligaclips and divided. The main splenic pedicle can be easily seen and secured with ligaclips or a vascular stapling device. Care should be taken to avoid damaging the tail of the pancreas, and the possibility of accessory spleens should be remembered. With precise attention to technique, complications should be minimal but may include intraoperative trauma (eg. diaphragmatic perforation), postoperative haemorrhage and basal lung consolidation (Targarona *et al*, 2000). Removal of the spleen may require an incision or it can be morcellated in a retrieval bag and sucked out where histology is not required (Park *et al*, 2000; Rosen *et al*, 2002).

Hernia repair

The first procedures for laparoscopic repair of inguinal and femoral hernia were carried out over ten years ago (Ger *et al*, 1990), and are now well established within the surgical armamentarium. The general principal involves placement of a mesh in the pre-peritoneal space thereby reinforcing the posterior wall of the inguinal canal deep to the abdominal wall musculature. There are two main approaches to the site of interest, namely the trans-abdominal pre-peritoneal (TAPP) and the totally extra-peritoneal (TEP) repair. *Figure 3.5* demonstrates the intra-abdominal view of the normal anatomical landmarks identified during a TAPP repair. An indirect hernia would be seen traversing the deep ring, whereas a direct hernia lies medial to this (*Figure 3.6*). Briefly, the TAPP approach involves access to the peritoneal cavity as in, for example, a laparoscopic cholecystectomy. The hernial site is identified, and the peritoneum above this is divided in a transverse line developing the pre-peritoneal space and reducing the hernia. The mesh is then placed into the pre-peritoneal space and the peritoneum closed. In the TEP repair the peritoneum is not breached. The first port is placed into the pre-peritoneal space and a 'pneumo-pre-peritoneum' is created. This then is the working space for the procedure, and the repair is carried out in a similar manner to the TAPP repair. Both approaches have their advocates and each has benefits and complications. In the final analysis it would appear that both are effective in treating the primary problem with minimal overall complications. A number of series comparing open and laparoscopic approach have reported essentially no difference between the two, except for reduced postoperative pain and reduced time to return to normal activities (The MRC laparoscopic groin hernia trial group, 1999; Bozuk *et al*, 2003; Andersson *et al*, 2003; McCormack *et al*, 2003). Some authorities recommend laparoscopic repair only in cases of bilateral or recurrent inguinal hernia (Gokalp *et al*, 2003; Nathan and Pappas, 2003) but these views have been challenged and many

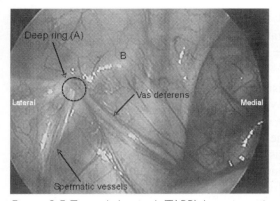

Figure 3.5: Transabdominal (TAPP) laparoscopic hernia repair. Intra-operative view of anatomical landmarks

centers are now performing the laparoscopic repair routinely. It is worth noting that an occult contralateral hernia is found in 30% of laparoscopic procedures; these can be repaired at the same time, thus removing the need for a subsequent operation. Femoral hernia is equally accessible to either of these two approaches and has been described with good outcome in the non-emergency presentation (Hernandez-Richter *et al*, 2000). Although the laparoscopic approach has been advocated even for obstructed inguinal and femoral hernia repair (Ferzli *et al*, 2004), this is not universally accepted at the present time in view of the risks of infection in the presence of a mesh, and secondary risk of bowel perforation with the use of mechanical instruments on potentially ischemic bowel.

The laparoscopic approach is now increasingly being used in repair of ventral hernias (both primary and secondary) (Heniford *et al*, 2003) and has been reported in the management of lumbar hernia (Arca *et al*, 1998; Sakarya *et al*, 2003).

In summary the increased availability of training in established laparoscopic centres has lead to a more widespread use of this approach in the repair of most common types of hernia. There are few contraindications to this type of surgery. They include the usual general surgical and anesthetic risks. The size of hernia is not as important as was once thought, and the repair of large inguinal scrotal hernias has been successfully carried out. Recurrence rates appear to be similar between open and laparoscopic repair (Lal *et al*, 2003) although most follow-up data is as yet short term only. Patient satisfaction appears to be greater in the laparoscopic group and this is most notable in patients who have undergone open hernia repair in the pre-laparoscopic era, and returned with a contralateral hernia which has been repaired laparoscopically. It is recommended that patients be offered the choice, which will to some extent be directed by accessibility to a laparoscopic unit.

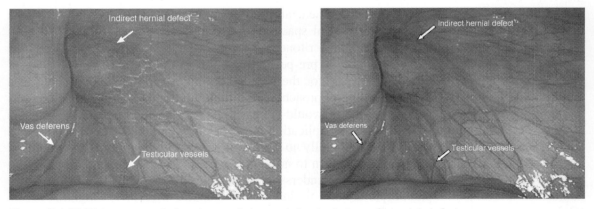

Figure 3.6: TAPP laparoscopic hernia repair. Intra-abdominal view of hernial defect

Current developments

Hand assisted laparoscopic surgery

Hand assisted laparoscopic surgery (HALS) has developed from the requirement for increased dexterity in prolonged or difficult procedures. This involves the creation of a mini-laparotomy and insertion of a plastic cushion device, which allows maintenance of the pneumoperitoneum whilst simultaneously providing access for the surgeon's hand to enter the peritoneal cavity and assist in the procedure (Glasgow and Swanstrom 2001; Romanelli *et al*, 2001). It has been used in a variety of operations, for example colectomy and gastric and esophageal cancer surgery, all of which may involve extensive lymphadenectomy and at times difficult mobilization. This approach is gaining popularity, with early studies showing favourable results (Usui *et al*, 2003; Tanimura *et al*, 2003).

Robotic surgery

In principle the mechanisms of this type of surgery have been explained elsewhere in this book, but suffice to say that robotic surgery is still under evaluation within the field of general surgery. It has been applied successfully to a number of different operations including cholecystectomy and colectomy. Most famously perhaps is the 'Lindbergh' operation undertaken by Professor Marescaux operating in New York on a patient in Strasbourg. In this instance one of the greatest obstacles to this particular operation was the telecommunication limitation with regard to signal transference across a great distance. Once this had been solved with high-speed data transfer (a transmission delay of only 150 milliseconds) the operation was then carried out successfully. This signals a new horizon for the laparoscopic surgeon. The future, in terms of operating at a site remote from the patient, has now been demonstrated by the successful completion of the Lindbergh operation. The remaining limitations will simply be a matter of technological refinement, financial viability and market forces.

Key points for *Chapter 3*

- Laparoscopic cholecystectomy is now the gold standard of treatment for gallstone disease with few absolute contraindications and performed increasingly as a daycase procedure.

- Common bile duct stones should be removed preoperatively by ERCP, but if found at surgery exploration of the duct can be safely performed laparoscopically.

- Laparoscopic fundoplication is indicated in severe acid reflux disease which persists despite maximal medical therapy and has a 90% success rate.

- Indications for bariatric surgery include clinical obesity for >5 years, dietary failure for at least one year, and age range 18–60.

- Current procedures include prosthetic gastric banding, gastric diversion and duodenal switch, where success is defined as ≥50% sustained reduction of excess weight.

- Laparoscopic colorectal surgery for both benign and malignant conditions is increasingly performed in specialist units, but only short-term survival data have been published.

- Laparoscopic adrenal surgery is indicated for benign lesions up to 15cm diameter.

- Control of functioning lesions must be achieved prior to surgery.

- Laparoscopic splenectomy is performed for benign tumours or cysts and haematological disorders.

- All types of hernia have been repaired laparoscopically, however it is most suited to bilateral and recurrent herniae.

References

Andersson B *et al* (2003) Laparoscopic extraperitoneal inguinal hernia repair versus open mesh repair: a prospective randomized controlled trial. *Surgery* **133(5):** 464–72

Anthuber M *et al* (2003) Outcome of laparoscopic surgery for rectal cancer in 101 patients. *Dis Colon Rectum* **46(8):** 1047–53

Arca MJ *et al* (1998) Laparoscopic repair of lumbar hernias. J Am Coll Surg. **187(2):** 147–52

Benotti PN *et al* (1989) Gastric restrictive operations for morbid obesity. *Am J Surg* **157(1):** 150–5

Berci GJ Sackier *et al* (1991) Routine or selected intraoperative cholangiography during laparoscopic cholecystectomy. *Am J Surg* **161:** 355–360

Bozuk M *et al* (2003) Disability and chronic pain after open mesh and laparoscopic inguinal hernia repair. *Am Surg* **69(10):** 839–41

Chevallier JM *et al* (2004) Complications after laparoscopic adjustable gastric banding for morbid obesity: experience with 1,000 patients over 7 years. *Obes Surg* **14(3):** 407–14

Chrysos E *et al* (2001) Prospective randomized trial comparing Nissen to Nissen-Rossetti technique for laparoscopic fundoplication. *Am J Surg* **182(3):** 215–21

Chung CC *et al* (2003) Laparoscopy and its current role in the management of colorectal disease. *Colorectal Dis* **5(6):** 528–43

Downs S *et al* (1996) Systematic review of the effectiveness and safety of laparoscopic cholecystectomy. *Annals R Coll Surg Eng* **78(3):** 241–323

Dunn, D *et al* (1994) Laparoscopic cholecystectomy in England and Wales: results of an audit by the Royal College of Surgeons of England. *Ann R Coll Surg Engl* **76(4):** 269–75

Ferzli G *et al* (2004) Laparoscopic extraperitoneal approach to acutely incarcerated inguinal hernia. *Surg Endosc* **18(2):** 228–31

Flum DR *et al* (2003) Intraoperative cholangiography and risk of common bile duct injury during cholecystectomy. *Jama* **289(13):** 1639–44

Gagner MA Lacroix *et al* (1992) Laparoscopic adrenalectomy in Cushing's syndrome and pheochromocytoma. *N Engl J Med* **327(14):** 1033

Ger R *et al* (1990) Management of indirect inguinal hernias by laparoscopic closure of the neck of the sac. *Am J Surg* **159(4):** 370–3

Glasgow RE, Swanstrom LL (2001) Hand-assisted gastroesophageal surgery. Semin *Laparosc Surg* **8(2):** 135–44

Gokalp A *et al* (2003) A prospective randomized study of Lichtenstein open tension-free versus laparoscopic totally extraperitoneal techniques for inguinal hernia repair. *Acta Chir Belg* **103(5):** 502–6

Granderath FA *et al* (2002) Long-term results of laparoscopic antireflux surgery. *Surg Endosc* **16(5):** 753–7

Guller U *et al* (2003) Laparoscopic *vs.* open colectomy: outcomes comparison based on large nationwide databases. *Arch Surg* **138(11):** 1179–86

Heniford BT *et al* (2003) Laparoscopic repair of ventral hernias: nine years' experience with 850 consecutive hernias. *Ann Surg* **238(3):** 391–9; discussion 399–400

Henry JF *et al* (2002) Results of laparoscopic adrenalectomy for large and potentially malignant tumors. *World J Surg* **26(8):** 1043–7

Hernandez-Richter T *et al* (2000) The femoral hernia: an ideal approach for the transabdominal preperitoneal technique (TAPP). *Surg Endosc* **14(8):** 736–40

Herron DM (2004) The surgical management of severe obesity. *Mt Sinai J Med* **71(1):** 63–71

Lacy AM *et al* (2002) Laparoscopy-assisted colectomy versus open colectomy for treatment of non-metastatic colon cancer: a randomised trial. *Lancet* **359(9325):** 2224–9

Lal P *et al* (2003) Randomized controlled study of laparoscopic total extraperitoneal versus open Lichtenstein inguinal hernia repair. *Surg Endosc* **17(6):** 850–6

Lee WJ *et al* (2004) Laparoscopic vertical banded gastroplasty and laparoscopic gastric bypass: a comparison. *Obes Surg* **14(5):** 626–34

Luketich JD *et al* (2003) Minimally invasive esophagectomy: outcomes in 222 patients. *Ann Surg* **238(4):** 486–94; discussion 494–5

McCormack K *et al* (2003) Laparoscopic techniques versus open techniques for inguinal hernia repair. *Cochrane Database Syst Rev* (1): CD001785

Moose D *et al* (2003) Laparoscopic Roux-en-Y gastric bypass: minimally invasive bariatric surgery for the superobese in the community hospital setting. *Am Surg* **69**(11): 930–2

Nathan JD and TN Pappas (2003), Inguinal hernia: an old condition with new solutions. *Ann Surg* **238**(6 Suppl): S148–57

Nguyen NT *et al* (2001) Minimally invasive Ivor Lewis esophagectomy. *Ann Thorac Surg* **72(2):** 593–6

Nguyen, NT *et al* (2003) Thoracoscopic and laparoscopic esophagectomy for benign and malignant disease: lessons learned from 46 consecutive procedures. *J Am Coll Surg* **197(6):** 902–13

O'Boyle CJ *et al* (2002) Division of short gastric vessels at laparoscopic nissen fundoplication: a prospective double-blind randomized trial with 5-year follow-up. *Ann Surg* **235(2):** 165–70

O'Brien PE and JB Dixon (2003) Lap-band: outcomes and results. *J Laparoendosc Adv Surg Tech A* **13(4):** 265–70

Park AG Birgisson *et al* (2000), Laparoscopic splenectomy: outcomes and lessons learned from over 200 cases. *Surgery* **126:** 660–667

Patankar SK *et al* (2003) Prospective comparison of laparoscopic vs. open resections for colorectal adenocarcinoma over a ten-year period. *Dis Colon Rectum* **46(5):** 601–11

Patel HR, Harris AM *et al* (2001) Adrenal masses: Management and investigation of adrenal incidentaloma. *Ann. R. Coll. Surg. Engl* **83:** 250–52

Ren CJ M Weiner *et al* (2004) Favorable early results of gastric banding for morbid obesity: the American experience. *Surg Endosc* **18(3):** 543–6

Richardson WS and JG Hunter (1999) Laparoscopic floppy Nissen fundoplication. *Am J Surg* **177(2):** 155–7

Romanelli JR, JJ Kelly *et al* (2001) Hand-assisted laparoscopic surgery in the United States: an overview. *Semin Laparosc Surg* **8(2):** 96–103

Rosen, M *et al* (2002) Outcome of laparoscopic splenectomy based on hematologic indication. *Surg Endosc* **16(2):** 272–9

Sakarya A *et al* (2003) Laparoscopic repair of acquired lumbar hernia. *Surg Endosc* **17(9):** 1494

Shimizu S *et al* (2003) Laparoscopic gastric surgery in a Japanese institution: analysis of the initial 100 procedures. *J Am Coll Surg* **197(3):** 372–8

Smith SC *et al* (2004) Open *vs.* laparoscopic Roux-en-Y gastric bypass: comparison of operative morbidity and mortality. *Obes Surg* **14(1):** 73–6

Tanimura, S *et al* (2003) Laparoscopic gastrectomy with regional lymph node dissection for upper gastric cancer. *Gastric Cancer* **6(1):** 64–8

Targarona EM *et al* (2000) Complications of laparoscopic splenectomy. *Arch Surg* **135(10):** 1137–40

The MRC Laparoscopic Groin Hernia Trial Group (1999) Laparoscopic versus open repair of groin hernia: a randomised comparison. *Lancet* **354(9174):** 185–90

Tsang WW, C.C. Chung *et al* (2003) Prospective evaluation of laparoscopic total mesorectal excision with colonic J-pouch reconstruction for mid and low rectal cancers. *Br J Surg* **90(7):** 867–71

Usui S *et al* (2003) Hand-assisted laparoscopic total gastrectomy for early gastric cancer. *Surg Laparosc Endosc Percutan Tech* **13(5):** 304–7

Weber DM (2003) Laparoscopic surgery: an excellent approach in elderly patients. *Arch Surg* **138(10):** 1083–8

Weber KJ *et al* (2003) Comparison of laparoscopic and open gastrectomy for malignant disease. Surg Endosc **17(6):** 968–71

Weeks JC *et al* (2002) Short-term quality-of-life outcomes following laparoscopic-assisted colectomy *vs* open colectomy for colon cancer: a randomized trial. *Jama* **287(3):** 321–8

Weiner RA *et al* (2004) Laparoscopic biliopancreatic diversion with duodenal switch: three different duodeno-ileal anastomotic techniques and initial experience. *Obes Surg* **14(3):** 334–40

Yamamoto S *et al* (2002) Prospective evaluation of laparoscopic surgery for rectosigmoidal and rectal carcinoma. *Dis Colon Rectum* **45(12):** 1648–54

CHAPTER 4

Minimally invasive treatments for benign and malignant prostatic disease

S Masood, C Kouriefs, M Arya, HRH Patel, JH Palmer

Benign Prostatic Hyperplasia (BPH) is a pathological process of ageing and the commonest urological condition of older men. BPH commonly presents with symptoms of bladder outflow obstruction for which up to 40% of men will undergo a surgical intervention. Since the first half of this century monopolar Transurethral resurection of the prostate (TURP) is the commonest and gold standard treatment for BPH. TURP has been around for many decades and has stood the test of time. The success of TURP is reported to be 80–95% and the re-treatment rate 8% at ten years. However, TURP carries significant morbidity and it is considered unsuitable for about 20% of patients in need of one. Several minimally invasive treatments have therefore emerged in the 1980s primarily aiming to provide as equally effective symptom relief as TURP but in a safer way.

The incidence of prostate cancer has more than doubled in the last ten years. There are multiple treatment options for localized prostate cancer but there is no consensus as to what constitutes appropriate treatment for any stage of disease, especially for localized cancers. Radical prostatectomy, radiation therapy, or watchful waiting all have their advocates. Scepticism about conventional treatments has stimulated patients and physicians to search for alternatives that are effective and associated with limited morbidity.

The different minimally invasive treatments for BPH and prostate cancer are reviewed in this chapter.

Introduction

Benign prostatic hyperplasia

BPH is the commonest urological condition in elderly men (McNaughton-Collins *et al*, 1999). About 50% of men aged 51–60 and 90% over ninety years of age have histological evidence of BPH (Carter and Coffey, 1990). Forty per cent of men with BPH will require surgical intervention for symptoms secondary to BPH at an average age of seventy-four years (Arrighi *et al*, 1991). In an ever ageing population the prevalence of BPH will continue to rise. BPH can be associated with Lower Urinary Tract Symptoms (LUTS) that impact on men's quality of life. The association between BPH and LUTS is complex. Fifty percent of men with BPH have LUTS (Roehrborn and McConnell, 2002). LUTS can be due to other lower urinary tract pathology than BPH. The 4th International Consultation for BPH has therefore recommended the use of the term LUTS instead of 'prostatism' (Denis *et al*, 1998). The American Urological Association guidelines (AUA) for the management of BPH state that only men with bothersome symptoms or complicated bladder outflow obstruction should be considered for active treatment options (AUA Guideline, 2003). The 'bother' from LUTS is very variable. In the past, people used to accept their LUTS as part of the ageing process and for fear of the available surgical options they used to suffer in silence. Prior to the introduction of TURP in the 1920s, open prostectomy was the gold standard treatment for BPH, either via the transvesical (Freyer's prostatectomy) or retropubic (Millin's prostatectomy) route. The introduction of fiberoptics by Karl Storz in 1959 and rod–lens endoscopes by Prof Hopkins (Reading University) made TURP a technically easier and safer surgical option and it remains the benchmark treatment of BPH and is the gold standard for comparison.

In the last twenty years a host of new, less invasive therapeutic options, appeared as possible competitors to TURP (*Table 4.1*). These new treatments are expected to be less costly per treatment episode, less time consuming and above all associated with less morbidity making them attractive to patients and clinicians. Since their introduction such treatments have had an impact on the way we manage BPH. Data from the 4th International Consultation on BPH suggests that the number of TURP performed in the USA has more than halved between 1987 (258000/ year) and 1997 (105000/ year) (Denis *et al*, 1998). Such decline is mirrored in Europe. In the UK, 33000 elective TURP were performed in 1999 compared to under 27000 in 2001. The new minimally invasive surgical option treatments are only partly to 'blame' for that decline as the introduction of more effective pharmacotherapy and phytotherapy have a major say in that. One should be careful of the initial overstaged success of new treatments. Are these minimally invasive surgical options for managing BPH as good competitors to TURP as some initially suggested? This chapter is aiming to review these procedures and provide the reader with a basic knowledge and understanding on which to base their BPH management decisions.

Table 4.1: Minimally invasive treatments for Benign Prostatic Hyperplasia (BPH)

A   Thermal based treatments
- Transurethral microwave thermotherapies (TUMT)
- Transurathral needle ablation (TUNA)
- LASER based treatments (VLAP, CLAP, HoLRP, HoLEP, ILC,KTP)
- Transurethral electrovaporization (TEVP)
- Transurethral incision of the prostate (TUIP/ BNI)
- High intensity focused ultrasound (HIFU)

B   Transurethral balloon dilatation of the prostate

C   Prostatic urethral endoprostheses
- Temporary biodegradable stents
- Permanent stents (Urolume, Memokath)

Prostate cancer

There is a dramatic increase in the number of patients diagnosed with prostate cancer in the last decade. In England and Wales prostate cancer is now the most frequently diagnosed cancer in men, excluding skin cancer, with 24725 prostate cancers diagnosed in 2000. In the USA prostate cancer incidence rates increased dramatically between 1988 and 1992 due to earlier diagnosis because of PSA blood testing. This incidence rate subsequently declined and then increased at a less rapid rate since 1995 due to increasing rate in men younger than sixty five (Cancer Facts and Figures, 2004).

The treatment of prostate cancer still remains controversial, and no consensus has been established as to what is the appropriate treatment for any stage of disease, especially for localized cancers. A significant number of men do not need intervention and can be safely kept under a 'watch and wait' policy. Traditionally men diagnosed with clinically localized prostate cancer had three treatment options: radical surgery, external beam radiotherapy and active surveillance (watch and wait). Radical prostatectomy and external beam radical radiotherapy are associated with considerable morbidity and hence many minimally invasive treatment options have emerged with some still in the experimental phase (*Table 4.4*). The aim of minimally invasive alternative treatment options should be equal efficacy, but a decrease in side effects.

Minimally invasive treatment for BPH

Medical (pharmacotherapy and phytotherapy) treatment as well as TURP are beyond the scope of this chapter. The rest of the minimal treatment options are discussed.

Thermal based treatments

Thermal based treatments utilize the effects of high temperatures on the prostatic tissue. Thermal based treatments achieving temperatures >45°C are referred to as 'thermotherapies' and those achieving temperatures <45°C are referred to as 'hyperthermias'. The latter group of treatments was explored first on animal prostate cancer cell lines and there was no demonstrable tissue effect. A meta-analysis by Matzkin (Matzkin, 1994) concluded that hyperthermia was not achieving sustained benefits on BPH management. This prompted the exploration of the effect of higher temperatures on the prostate (Thermotherapies). Such temperatures result in prostate denervation and autonomic receptor (adrenoceptors-α) destruction as well as reduced prostatic volume by coagulative necrosis and subsequent sloughing of the necrotic tissue.

Transurethral Microwave Thermotherapy (TUMT)

TUMT (*Figure 4.1*) uses microwaves to generate the necessary therapeutic temperatures. It is the most popular minimally invasive treatment and this is reflected by the abundance of

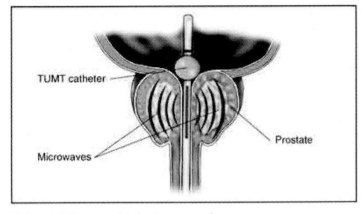

Figure 4.1: Transurethral microwave therapy

recent publications on the subject. It was first studied under an FDA approved protocol in 1991 and five years later it received final FDA approval. At present there are several TUMT devices which differ in the amount of energy output, cooling system, treatment time and the way the desired effect is monitored. Such devices include the high-energy (HE) Prostatron, Targis and ProstLund and the low-energy (LE) TherMatrx and Urowave.

Several randomized controlled trials have shown significantly better improvements when treating BPH with TUMT compared to Sham procedures (De Wildt *et al*, 1996; Blute *et al*, 1996; Brehmer *et al*, 1999). There are no comparative studies to confirm superiority of one device over another. However, there is evidence to suggest that HE devices provide more substantial and sustained improvements in symptom scores, urine flow rate and bladder emptying (Gravas *et al*, 2003). Tsai *et al* (Tsai *et al*, 2001) in a retrospective review of forty-five men with BPH, treated with LE-TUMT, reported an 84% additional treatment rate at five years of follow-up (*Table 4.2*). On the other hand, Floratos *et al* (Floratos *et al*, 2001) reported a Randomized Prospective Trial (RCT) comparing HE-TUMT to TURP and found an additional treatment rate of 22% after HE-TUMT compared to a 13% following TURP at three years follow-up (*Table 4.3*).

The main advantage of TUMT like other minimally invasive treatments is reduced morbidity. In a RCT comparing TURP to TUMT, Wagrell *et al*, (Wagrell *et al*, 2002) reported a 17% TURP-related significant morbidity rate compared to 2% following TUMT. Significant unexpected injuries have been reported following TUMT and clinicians are strongly advised to adhere to the safety recommendations published by FDA (FDA/CDRH, 2003). Most importantly regional or general (GA) anesthesia should be avoided because pain is an important safety mechanism in avoiding unwanted destruction of tissues. The ability to perform TUMT without GA or regional anaesthesia on an outpatient basis adds to its economic advantages.

TransUrethral Needle Ablation of the prostate (TUNA)

TUNA (*Figure 4.2*) involves heating and ablating the prostate using low level radiofrequency waves (490KHz). The energy is delivered by two 18-gauge needles through a specially designed catheter that resembles a cystoscope. The two needles are deployed at the tip of the catheter and pierce the prostatic urothelium entering the hyperplastic prostatic adenoma. Temperatures of about 100°C are aimed for coagulative necrosis to occur.

Cimentepe *et al* (Cimentepe *et al*, 2003), compared TUNA to TURP in a randomized controlled trial. TUNA was reported to be an effective treatment with significant improvement in flow rate and IPSS score but the improvement was less than TURP (*Table 4.3*). What is most important is the high re-operation rate reported in the literature within two years of treatment

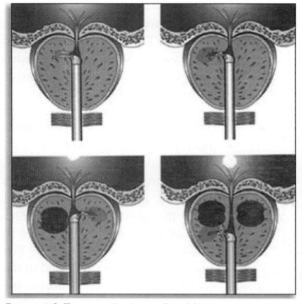

Figure 4.2: Transurethral needle ablation

(10–15%) and up to 30% at five years (*Table 4.2*) (Zlotta *et al*, 2003). TUNA is performed under regional or general anesthetic.

LASER based treatments

LASER is a form of energy and not a treatment. Broad terms such as 'laser prostatectomy' or 'laser treatment' are best avoided because different lasers interact with the prostatic tissue in different ways. The characteristics of the interaction is dependent on the wavelength, power and type of emission (pulsed or continuous). Lasers can resect, vaporize or coagulate prostatic tissue or even work in a combination of ways (laser hybrids). The most commonly used lasers in urology are Nd-YAG (neodymium:yttrium-aluminium-garnet) and Ho-YAG (Holmium: yttrium-aluminium-garnet). Nd-YAG has a shorter wavelength (λ=1060nm) than Ho-YAG laser (λ=2140nm). The later therefore has poor penetration (0.04mm) compared to the deeper penetration of Nd-YAG (0.5–1.75cm).

Techniques

Visual Laser Ablation of Prostate (VLAP)

This technique (*Figure 4.3*) was first described by Costello *et al* in 1992 (Costello *et al*, 1992). It utilizes Nd-YAG laser in a non-contact mode. The laser fiber is held a short distance (2mm) from the prostatic tissue under cystoscopic vision. This results in deep thermal coagulative necrosis and eventual sloughing of the prostatic adenoma within six to eight weeks. It is a popular technique amongst urologists because of its sharp learning curve. The AUA guidelines on BPH report it to be an effective treatment option. They however emphasise a high rate of post-operative urinary retention (21%) compared to 5% after TURP and a high incidence of early irritative LUTS.

Intermediate follow-up clinical trials on VLAP are now available. Sengor *et al* (Sengor *et al*, 2002) report sustained symptom improvement at three years follow-up and a re-operation rate of 5.5% (*Table 4.2*).

Contact Laser Ablation of the Prostate (CLAP)

This is a less popular technique. It utilizes Nd-YAG in a contact mode. That results in higher tissue energy and temperatures than VLAP resulting in vaporization of the prostatic tissue and immediate channel, like TURP. CLAP is a more cumbersome technique.

Early results up to two years are similar to VLAP but intermediate follow-up studies suggest a significantly higher re-operation rate (23%) (Bryan *et al*, 2000; Keoghane *et al*, 2000). The Oxford Laser Trial using a high-powered Nd-YAG contact tip, reported an 18% re-operation rate at five years follow-up (Keoghane *et al*, 2000).

Holmium Laser Resection of the Prostate (HoLRP)

This procedure has a longer learning curve but once mastered it seems to produce good early and intermediate results. Gilling *et al* (Gilling *et al*, 2000) published a RCT comparing HoLRP and TURP (*Table 4.3*). They reported equal results at two years follow-up. The same group presented the four years follow-up results at the AUA 2002 annual meeting (Gilling, 2002). Improvements after HoLRP were sustained and the re-operation rate was equal to that of TURP.

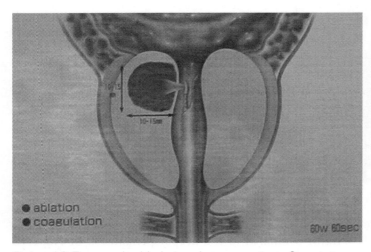

Figure 4.3: *Transurethral holmium laser resection of prostate*

Holmium Laser Enucleation of the Prostate (HoLEP)

This technique adapts the concept of open prostatectomy which is to enucleate the prostatic adenoma from the compressed peripheral zone of the prostate, also referred to as the surgical capsule. The large adenoma is morcellated in the bladder and extracted through the cystoscope. HoLEP holds promise for the future.

There is a lack of long-term follow-up studies but HoLEP is reported to provide equal results

Table 4.2: Summary of retrospective and prospective studies assessing the efficacy of minimally invasive treatments for BPH

Study/ Year	Cohort	Treatment	Follow up (months)	Additional/ re-treatment rate
Gravas *et al* 2003	41	HE-TUMT	12	NA
Tsai *et al* 2001	65	LE-TUMT	49	84%
Floratos *et al* 2000	41	HE-TUMT	12	25%
Floratos *et al* 2000	107	VLAP	53	14%
	30	CLAP	47	14%
	53	ILC	34	41%
Zlotta *et al* 2003	188	TUNA	63	15%
Sengor *et al* 2002	230	VLAP	36	5.5%
Knoll *et al* 2003	72	ILC	84	30%
Sirls *et al* 1994	41	TUIP	53	NA
Sullivan *et al* 1999	46	HIFU	12	30%
Madersbacher *et al* 2000	98	HIFU	41	44%
Masood *et al* 2004	62	Urolume	144	48%

to TURP at shortterm follow-up (*Table 4.3*) (Tan *et al*, 2003). Re-operation, stricture and incontinence rates are equal to TURP. HoLEP has been used in large prostates. Gilling *et al* (Gilling *et al*, 2000) and Hettiarachchi *et al* (Hettiarachchi *et al*, 2002) reported successful results in treating prostates in excess of 100g with no risk of TUR syndrome and minimal bleeding. Moody and Lingeman (Moody and Lingeman, 2001) compared HoLEP to open prostatectomy in a retrospective and Kuntz and Lehrich (Kuntz and Lehrich, 2002) in a prospective study. They both reported comparable improvements. HoLEP had lower postoperative morbidity and hospital stay. The later series reported a shorter operating time in the open prostatectomy group. An important advantage of HoLEP

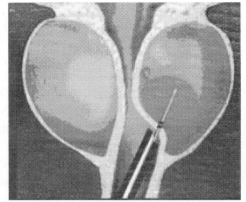

Figure 4.4: Interstitial laser coagulation

compared to other laser techniques is that it allows for histological examination. A recent study by Naspro *et al* (Naspro *et al*, 2004) showed no compromise in the detection of carcinoma of the prostate when comparing TURP and HoLEP resected specimens.

Interstitial laser coagulation

This procedure (*Figure 4.4*) involves the insertion of the laser fiber into the prostatic adenoma resulting in coagulative necrosis and subsequent sloughing of the adenoma. Knoll *et al* (Knoll *et al*, 2003) reported a seven years follow-up clinical trial on treating thirty-four patients with ILC. The re-operation rate was 15% and another 15% were started on medical BPH therapies (*Table 4.2*).

KTP laser prostatectomy

KTP (Potassium Titanyl Phospate) laser is effective in cutting and vaporizing the prostate. In-vivo studies have shown superior coagulative/hemostatic properties to conventional monopolar

Table 4.3: Summary of retrospective and prospective studies assessing the efficacy of minimally invasive treatments for BPH

Study/Year	Cohort	Treatment	Follow up months	Difference
Floratos *et al* 2001	155	HE-TUMT	33	NS
Wagnell *et al* 2002	154	HE-TUMT	12	NS
Cimentepe *et al* 2003	59	TUNA	18	NS
Hill *et al* 2004	121	TUNA	60	NS
Keoghane *et al* 2000	57	CLAP	60	NS
Tan *et al* 2003	61	HoLEP	12	NS
Gilling *et al* 2000	120	HoLRP	24	NS
Tkocz *et al* 2002	100	TUIP	24	NS
Riehmann *et al* 1995	120	TUIP	34	NS

NS – no statistically significant difference in the symptomatic improvement after each treatment, although some studies have shown a trend towards higher improvement with TURP

TURP (Reich *et al*, 2004). Another advantage of KTP laser is instantaneous vaporization of prostatic tissue which allows for early removal of the catheter in contrast to Nd-YAG laser prostatectomies where late tissue sloughing requires prolonged catheterization. Like other laser treatments there is lack of long-term data on KTP prostatectomy but in the short-term it appears to produce symptomatic improvement comparable to TURP. Carter *et al* (Carter *et al*, 1999) and Shingleton *et al* (Shingleton *et al*, 1999) demonstrated equivalent decrease in symptom score (AUA International Prostate Symptom Score (IPSS)) and increase in maximum urine flow rate at twelve months follow-up. A more recent prospective single-arm trial on KTP laser prostatectomy, with twelve months follow-up, showed encouraging results (Te *et al*, 2004). The AUA symptom score improved significantly from twenty-four before treatment to 4.3 after treatment. Significant improvements were reported in maximum urine flow (7.8ml/s pre- and 22.6 ml/s post-treatment) as well as in the post-void residual urine volume (114 *vs*. 24.8ml) (Te *et al*, 2004). Once again long-term data is awaited from KTP which alongside Holmium laser prostatectomies hold great promise and appear to be good competitors for conventional monopolar TURP.

Transurethral Electrovaporisation of the Prostate (TEVP)

This procedure adapts an old device into a new concept. The old device is the roller-ball used towards the end of TURP for hemostasis. The roller-ball is run along the prostate using a high-energy cutting current. This results in prostate ablation and a cavity formation. Recently thick vaporizing loops have been developed through which vaporization and resection of the prostate can be done at the same time. Kaplan and Te described this procedure in 1995 (Kaplan and Te, 1995). They studied twenty-five men with moderate bladder outflow obstruction (BOO) symptoms and found an improvement in symptom score (from 17.8 to 4.2) and maximum flow rate (from 7.4 to17.3 ml/sec) at three months. Postoperative irritative LUTS and urinary retention (AUR) appear to be higher than with TURP. Evidence of sustained long-term results is lacking.

Transurethral Incision of the Prostate (TUIP)

This is an endoscopic technique mainly used for younger patients with small prostates (<30gr). Using a conventional resectoscope and Collings knife the prostate is incised from near the ureteric orifices to the veromentanum. Commonly two incisions are made at 5 and 7 o'clock although some urologists do one incision at 6 o'clock. Sirls *et al* (Sirls *et al*, 1994) reported urodynamically proven improvements sustained at fifty-three months of follow-up (*Table 4.2*). The main advantage of TUIP over TURP is a lower risk for retrograde ejaculation (15–20%).

High Intensity Focused Ultrasound (HIFU)

HIFU uses high frequency and intensity focused ultrasounds to achieve intraprostatic temperatures of about 70°C and once again result in coagulative necrosis of the prostate.

There is lack of long-term follow-up clinical trials. Sullivan *et al* (Sullivan *et al*, 1999) published the Canadian experience in treating forty-six patients with BPH in three different institutions. Although they report HIFU to be an effective procedure, the symptom improvement appears to be inferior to TURP at one year. They also report a high re-operation rate of 30%. Madersbacher *et al* (Madersbacher *et al,* 2000) report a re-operation rate of 44% at a mean follow-up of forty-one months (*Table 4.2*). AUA guidelines on the management of BPH advise that HIFU is still on its investigational stage and it should not be offered outside the framework of clinical trials (AUA Guideline, 2003).

Transurethral balloon dilatation of prostate

Prostatic dilatation is performed by an especially designed balloon which is inflated in the prostatic urethra endoscopically. It was used for small prostates and has very few complications. Initial enthusiasm died very soon when disappointing results were reported (Lepor *et al*, 1992). AUA guidelines do not recommend this as a treatment option for BPH (AUA Guideline, 2003).

Prostatic urethral endoprostheses (prostatic stents)

The concept of stents in medicine is not new; it has been used in cardiovascular and gastrointestinal pathologies. Fabian first described the use of 'urological spiral', a temporary stent, in treating BPH, in 1980 (Fabian, 1980). These devices are implanted endoscopically in the prostatic urethra. The aim is to keep the prostatic urethra patent and hence relieve prostatic obstruction. The stents can be either temporary or permanent

Temporary and biodegradable stents

These stents are tubular devices that are made of either a non-absorbable or a biodegradable material. Temporary stents can be left in-situ for up to three years and then can be removed. They neither become covered by the urethral epithelium nor become incorporated into the urethral wall. Memokath; a temporary stent has been successfully used by Poulsen *et al* (Poulsen *et al*, 1993).

The biodegradable stents slowly break down and are excreted via the urethra spontaneously after some time. These stents have been used after various procedures like microwave thermotherapy and laser therapy with variable results.

Permanent stents

The permanent stents were initially used for the treatment of recurrent urethral strictures; its role was later extended to treat BPH and detrusor sphincter dyssynergia (DSD). The Urolume endoprosthesis (American Medical Systems, Minnetonka, Minn) (*Figure 4.5*) is the most commonly used permanent stent. Oesterling *et al* (Oesterling *et al*, 1994) from USA reported a multicentre trial and Guazzoni *et al* (Guazzoni *et al*, 1994) conducted a European study for the use of Urolume in BPH and showed promising results at two years of follow-up but associated with a high explantation rate. In the authors' experience with Urolume, there was a significant improvement in symptoms after five years (Anjum *et al*, 1997), although at twelve years of follow-up (Masood *et al*, 2004) the explantation rate is 48%, most of which are removed in the first two years

In March 2005 after successfully treating more then 7000 patients with HIFU, a European HIFU club has been launched to support this new technology. The aim of the club is to share clinical experience and knowledge within the urologist community. In the UK NICE (National Institute of Clinical Excellence) has recently approved the use of HIFU for the treatment of prostate cancer either as primary or salvage therapy.

Cryosurgery

Cryosurgery is a treatment modality that uses a technique to selectively freeze tissue and thereby cause controlled tissue destruction. The procedure involves placement of multiple small diameter probes through the perineum into the prostate tissue at selected spatial intervals. Transrectal ultrasound is used to properly position the cylindrical probes before activation of the liquid Argon cooling element, which lowers the tissue temperature below minus 40 degrees Centigrade.

The results of first, second and third generation of cryosurgery are now available.

Long term follow-up study was performed by Bahn *et al* (Bahn *et al*, 2002) who assessed 590 patients where cryosurgery was used as primary therapy for localized or locally advanced prostate cancer. Patients were stratified into three risk groups according to clinical characteristics, and the mean follow-up for all patients was 5.4 years. Using a PSA-based definition of biochemical failure (of 0.5 ng/mL), the seven-year actuarial biochemical disease-free survivals for low, medium and high-risk patients were 61%, 68% and 61%, respectively.

Brachytherapy

Brachytherapy involves insertion of a radioactive source directly into the prostate gland, allowing a high dose of radiation to be delivered over a short distance around the source, sparing normal tissue. Two types are used in the treatment of localized prostate cancer: iodine-125 seeds or palladium-103, as a permanent low dose implant and iridium-192 as a temporary, high dose implant used in conjunction with External Beam Radiotherapy (EBRT).

A randomized study comparing radical prostatectomy, external beam radiation therapy and brachytherapy has not been done. Potters *et al* reported (Potters *et al*, 2004) on 1819 patients with T1 and T2 adenocarcinoma of the prostate. These patients received monotherapy treatment without additional adjuvant therapy. External beam radiotherapy was given to 340 patients, 746 had radical prostatectomy whereas 733 received permanent prostate brachytherapy. As in other studies pre-treatment PSA (Prostate Specific Antigen) levels, and biopsy Gleason score determined outcome. Biochemical failure rates were found to be similar between brachytherapy, radical prostatectomy and external beam radiotherapy as monotherapy for clinically localized prostate cancer.

Potters *et al* (Potters *et al*, 2005) have also shown that in patients with localized prostate carcinoma, permanent prostate brachytherapy has acceptable freedom from biochemical recurrence in the long term (twelve years).

Long-term follow-up of PSA data and survival are necessary before any conclusions can be made about the efficacy of minimally invasive options.

Key points – *Minimally Invasive Treatment for Prostate Cancer*

- Most of the minimally invasive treatment options are still in experimental stages.
- HIFU has been approved by NICE for the treatment of prostate cancer either as primary or salvage therapy. The negative biopsy rate has been reported in up to 93% of the patients following HIFU.
- Cryotherapy is often reported as a salvage procedure after failed conventional treatments but has been used successfully for primary localized prostate cancer.
- Long term results with brachytherapy demonstrate over 90% of low risk prostate cancer patients, disease free at 10 years.
- Long-term follow-up of PSA data and survival are necessary before any conclusions can be made about the efficacy of minimally invasive options.

References

American Cancer Society (2004) Cancer Facts and Figures 2004 *http://www.cancer.org/downloads/STT/CAFF_finalPWsecured.pdf*

Anjum MI, Chari R *et al* (1997) Long-term clinical results and quality of life after insertion of a self-expanding flexible endourethral prosthesis. *B J Urol* **80(6):** 885–8

Anjum MI, Palmer JH (1995). A technique for removal of the Urolume endourethral wallstent prosthesis. *Br J Urol* **76(5):** 655–6

Arrighi HM, Metter EJ *et al* (1991) Natural history of benign prostatic hyperplasia and risk of prostatectomy. The Baltimore Longitudinal Study of Aging. *Urology* **38(Suppl 1):** 4–8

AUA Guideline on Management of Benign Prostatic Hyperplasia (2003). Chapter 1: Diagnosis and Treatment Recommendations. *J Urol* **170(2, Part 1):** 530–547, August 2003

Bahn DK, Lee F *et al* (2002) Targeted cryoablation of the prostate: 7 year outcomes in the primary treatment of prostate cancer. *Urology* **60(2 suppl 1):** 3–11

Blana A, Walter B *et al* (2004) High-intensity focused ultrasound for the treatment of localized prostate cancer: 5 year experience. *Urology* **63(2):** 297–300

Blute ML, Patterson DE *et al* (1996) Transurethral microwave thermotherapy *vs.* sham treatment: double-blind randomized study. *J Endourol* **10(6):** 565–73.

Brehmer M, Wiksell H *et al* (1999) Sham treatment compared with 30 or 60 min of thermotherapy for benign prostatic hyperplasia: a randomized study. *BJU Int* **84(3):** 292–6

Bryan NP, Hastie KJ *et al* (2000) Randomised prospective trial of contact laser prostatectomy (CLAP) versus visual laser coagulation of the prostate (VLAP) for the treatment of benign prostatic hyperplasia. 2-year follow-up. *Eur Urol* **38(3):** 265–71.

Carter A, Sells H *et al* (1999) A prospective randomized controlled trial of hybrid laser treatment or transurethral resection of the prostate, with a 1 year follow-up. *BJU Int* **83:** 254–59.

Carter HB, Coffey DS (1990) The prostate: An increasing medical problem. *Prostate* **16:** 39–48

Cimentepe E, Unsal A *et al* (2003) Randomized clinical trial comparing transurethral needle ablation with transurethral resection of the prostate for the treatment of benign prostatic hyperplasia: results at 18 months. *J Endourol* **17(2):** 103–7.

Costello AJ, Bowsher WG *et al* (1992) Laser ablation of the prostate in patients with benign prostatic hypertrophy. *Br J Urol* **69(6):** 603–8.

De Wildt MJ, Hubregtse M *et al* (1996) A 12-month study of the placebo effect in transurethral microwave thermotherapy. *Br J Urol* **77(2):** 221–7.

Denis L, McConnell J *et al* (1998) Recommendations of the International Scientific Committee: the evaluation and treatment of lower urinary tract symptoms (LUTS) suggestive of benign prostatic obstruction. In: Proceedings of the 4th International Consultation on Benign Prostatic Hyperplasia. Edited by L Denis, K Griffiths, S Khoury, ATK McDonnell, C Chatelain *et al*. United Kingdom: Plymbridge Distributors, ltd., 669–684

Fabian KM (1980) Der intraprostatische "Partielle Katheter" (urologische spiral). *Urologe* [A] **19:** 236

FDA/Center for Devices and Radiological Health (CDRH) resources page. US Food and Drug Administration Website. Available at: *http://www.fda.gov/cdrh/pdf/P000043b.pdf.* (Accessed January 15, 2003)

Floratos DL, Kiemeney LA *et al* (2001) Long-term follow up of randomized transurethral microwave thermotherapy versus transurethral prostatic resection study. *J Urol* **165(5):** 1533–8.

Floratos DL, Sonke GS *et al* (2000) Long-term follow-up of laser treatment for lower urinary tract symptoms suggestive of bladder outlet obstruction. *Urology* **56(4):** 604–9

Floratos DL, Sonke GS *et al* (2000) High energy transurethral microwave thermotherapy for the treatment of patients in urinary retention. *J Urol* **163(5):** 1457–60

Gilling P (2002). Holmium laser resection *vs.* TURP (abstract). In: abstracts of the AUA, Orlando 2002. *J Urol* **167**(suppl): 1158

Gilling PJ, Kennett KM *et al* (2000) Holmium laser enucleation of the prostate for glands larger than 100 g: an endourologic alternative to open prostatectomy. *J Endourol* **14(6):** 529–31.

Gilling PJ, Kennett KM *et al* (2000) Holmium laser resection vs transurethral resection of the prostate: results of a randomized trial with 2 years of follow-up. *J Endourol* **14(9):** 757–60.

Gravas S, Laguna P *et al* (2003) Thermotherapy and thermoablation for benign prostatic hyperplasia. *Curr Opin Urol* **13(1):** 45–9.

Guazzoni G, Montorsi F *et al* (1994) A modified prostatic UroLume Wallstent for healthy patients with symptomatic benign prostatic hyperplasia: a European Multicenter Study. *Urology* **44(3):** 364–70

Hankey BF, Feuer EJ *et al* (1999). Cancer surveillance series: interpreting trends in prostate cancer- part 1: evidence of the facts of screening in recent prostate cancer incidence, mortality and survival rates. *J Nat Cancer Inst* **91:** 1017–1024

Hettiarachchi JA, Samadi AA *et al* (2002) Holmium laser enucleation for large (greater than 100 mL) prostate glands. *Int J Urol* **9(5):** 233–6

Hill B, Belville W *et al* (2004) Transurethral needle ablation versus transurethral resection of the prostate for the treatment of symptomatic benign prostatic hyperplasia: 5-year results of a prospective, randomized, multicenter clinical trial. *J Urol* **171(6):** 2336–40

Kaplan SA, Te AE (1995) Transurethral electrovaporization of the prostate: a novel method for treating men with benign prostatic hyperplasia. *Urology* **45(4):** 566–72

Keoghane SR, Sullivan ME *et al* (2000) Five-year data from the Oxford Laser Prostatectomy Trial. *BJU Int* **86(3):** 227–8

Knoll T, Michel MS *et al* (2003) Long-term follow-up of interstitial laser coagulation in the treatment of benign prostatic hyperplasia. *Aktuelle Urol* **34(1):** 48–51

Kuntz RM, Lehrich K (2002) Transurethral holmium laser enucleation versus transvesical open enucleation for prostate adenoma greater than 100 gm: a randomized prospective trial of 120 patients. *J Urol* **168(4 Pt 1):** 1465–9

Lepor H, Sypherd D *et al* (1992) Randomized double-blind study comparing the effectiveness of balloon dilatation of the prostate and cystoscopy for the treatment of symptomatic benign prostatic hyperplasia. *J Urol* **147(3):** 639–42

Madersbacher S, Schatzl G *et al* (2000) Long-term outcome of transrectal high- intensity focused ultrasound therapy for benign prostatic hyperplasia. *Eur Urol* **37(6):** 687–94

Masood S, Djaladat H *et al* (2004) The 12 year outcome analysis of an endourethral Wallstent for treating benign prostatic hyperplasia. *BJU Int* **94(9):** 1271–4

Matzkin, H (1994) Hyperthermia as a treatment modality in benign prostatic hyperplasia. *Urology* **43:** 17

McNaughton-Collins M, Stafford RS *et al* (1999) Distinguishing chronic prostatitis and benign prostatic hyperplasia symptoms: Results of a national survey of physician visits. *Urology* **53:** 921–925

Moody JA, Lingeman JE (2001) Holmium laser enucleation for prostate adenoma greater than 100 gm comparison to open prostatectomy. *J Urol* **165(2):** 459–62

Naspro R, Freschi M *et al* (2004) Holmium laser enucleation versus transurethral resection of the prostate. Are histological findings comparable? *J Urol* **171(3):** 1203–6

Oesterling JE, Kaplan SA *et al* (1994) The North American experience with the UroLume endoprosthesis as a treatment for benign prostatic hyperplasia: Long-term results. The North American UroLume Study Group. *Urology* **44:** 353–362

Potters L, Klein EA *et al* (2004) Monotherapy for stage T1-T2 prostate cancer: radical prostatectomy, external beam radiotherapy, or permanent seed implantation. *Radiother Oncol* **71(1):** 29–33

Potters L, Morgenstern C *et al* (2005) 12 year outcomes following permanent prostate brachytherapy in patients with clinically localized prostate cancer. *J Urol* **173(5):** 1562–6

Poulsen AL, Shou J *et al* (1993) Memokath: a second generation of intraprostatic spirals. *Br J Urol* **72:** 331–37

Reich O, Bachmann A *et al* (2004) Experimental comparison of high power (80W) potassium titanyl phospate laser vaporization and transurethral resection of the prostate. *J Urol* **171:** 2502–4

Riehmann M, Knes JM *et al* (1995) Transurethral resection versus incision of the prostate: a randomized, prospective study. *Urology* **45(5):** 768–75

Roehrborn CG, McConnell JD (2002) Etiology, pathophysiology, epidemiology and natural history of benign prostatic hyperplasia. In: *Campbell's Urology*, 8th ed Walsh PC, Retik AB, Vaughan ED, Jr Wein AJ (eds). Philadelphia, WB Saunders 1297–1330

Sengor F, Gurdal M *et al* (2002) Neodymium:YAG visual laser ablation of the prostate: 7 years of experience with 230 patients. *J Urol* **167(1):** 184–7

Shingleton WB, Terrell F *et al* (1999) A randomized prospective study of laser ablation of the prostate versus transurethral resection of the prostate in men with benign prostatic hyperplasia. *Urology* **54(6):** 1017–21

Sirls T, Ganabathi K *et al* (1994) Transurethral incision of the prostate: an objective and subjective evaluation of long-term efficacy *J Urol* (Paris) **100(5):** 249–56

Sullivan L, Casey RW *et al* (1999) Canadian experience with high intensity focused ultrasound for the treatment of BPH. *Can J Urol* **6(3):** 799–805

Tan AH, Gilling PJ *et al* (2003) A randomized trial comparing holmium laser enucleation of the prostate with transurethral resection of the prostate for the treatment of bladder outlet obstruction secondary to benign prostatic hyperplasia in large glands (40 to 200 grams). *J Urol* **170(4 Pt 1):** 1270–4

Te AE, Malloy TR *et al* (2004) Photoselective vaporization of the prostate for the treatment of benign prostatic hyperplasia: 12-month results from the first United States multicenter prospective trial. *J Urol* **172(4 Pt 1):** 1404–8

Thurroff S, Chaussy C *et al* (2003) High-intensity focused ultrasound and localized prostate cancer: efficacy results from the European multicentric study. *J Endourol* **17(8):** 673–7

Tkocz M, Prajsner A (2002) Comparison of long-term results of transurethral incision of the prostate with transurethral resection of the prostate, in patients with benign prostatic hypertrophy. *Neurourol Urodyn* **21(2):** 112–6

Tsai YS, Lin JS *et al* (2001) Transurethral microwave thermotherapy for symptomatic benign prostatic hyperplasia: long-term durability with Prostcare. *Eur Urol* **39(6):** 688-92; discussion 693–4

Wagrell L, Schelin S *et al* (2002) Feedback microwave thermotherapy versus TURP for clinical BPH--a randomized controlled multicenter study. *Urology* **60(2):** 292–9

Zlotta AR, Giannakopoulos X *et al* (2003) Long-term evaluation of transurethral needle ablation of the prostate for treatment of symptomatic benign prostatic hyperplasia: clinical outcome up to five years from three centers. *Eur Urol* **44(1):** 89–93

CHAPTER 5

Percutaneous surgery (benign and malignant) renal disease

AJ Young, PL Acher, HRH Patel, RA Miller

Since the first percutaneous nephrolithotomy (PCNL) almost thirty years ago, percutaneous surgery has evolved to encompass a wide range of procedures. Percutaneous access can be gained either antegrade or retrograde, a bleeding diathesis being the major contraindication to either approach.

Diagnostic applications include antegrade pyelography and pressure-perfusion studies. Therapeutic applications include nephrostomy drainage, antegrade ureteric stenting, balloon dilation and endoureterotomy for ureteric strictures, endopyelotomy, endopyeloplasty, and dismembered pyeloplasty for UPJ obstruction, PCNL, resection of low grade upper tract transitional cell carcinoma and finally percutaneous radiofrequency or cryoablation for renal cell carcinoma lesions that are not suitable for surgical resection.

Complications from percutaneous surgery arise from the tract (eg. hemorrhage, renal and surrounding structure damage), and from the procedure performed. These should however be considered in relation to the morbidity of the open surgical procedures that percutaneous intervention has replaced.

Introduction

The first percutaneous nephrostomy was recorded in 1865, but it was not until 1976 that percutaneous nephrolithotomy (PCNL) was described (Fernstrom and Johansson, 1976). Since then percutaneous renal surgery has evolved greatly, its role being constantly redefined in response to new technology (eg. extracorporeal shock wave lithotripsy (ESWL) and flexible ureteroscopy) and advanced surgical techniques (eg. laparoscopic surgery). However it remains a core technique for the modern surgeon in dealing with both benign and more recently malignant conditions of the upper urinary tract.

Gradually the scope of procedures that can be performed via percutaneous access has been expanded to include antegrade endopyelotomy (Ramsay *et al*, 1984), resection of upper tract transitional cell carcinoma (TCC) (Tomera *et al*, 1982) and more recently dismembered pyeloplasty (Sharp *et al*, 2003). In addition to this one of the most exciting evolving areas in percutaneous surgery involves the use of radiofrequency and cryoablation techniques for the treatment of renal tumours.

The aim of this chapter is to provide a summary of the principles underpinning percutaneous surgery as well as discuss the latest developments and applications.

AJ Young, PL Acher, HRH Patel, RA Miller

Principles of percutaneous surgery

Access

Percutaneous access to the kidney can be gained by either antegrade (LeRoy, 1996) or retrograde (Hosking, 1996) approaches. The antegrade approach is more commonly used as it offers accurate positioning of the tract and the potential for multiple renal punctures without having to reposition the patient. The retrograde approach is favoured by some authors, especially for hypermobile or malrotated/positioned kidneys although is less suitable for lower pole tracts. Originally two systems were available for retrograde tracts, the Lawson or Hawkins-Hunter; however due to lack of use the Hawkins-Hunter system has recently been discontinued. Detailed descriptions of these procedures can be found elsewhere (LeRoy, 1996; Hosking, 1996). The principles of establishing a surgical percutaneous tract include:

Antegrade tract
- Normal clotting studies must be established.
- Placement of a ureteric catheter. This allows retrograde injection of contrast media which opacifies the collecting system prior to puncture. This can be stained blue to aid identification of successful entry into the collecting system.
- Patient positioning. The patient is placed prone on the operating table with appropriate padding and support.
- Puncture site is selected. A posterior calyx is preferred as this reduces the chance of vascular injury. The ideal site is the shortest tract below the twelfth rib to the calyx. However for various reasons a mid or upper pole puncture may be required, in which case a supra-twelve or supra-eleven puncture may be appropriate. The puncture site is marked with a hemostat.
- Needle puncture. This proceeds under fluoroscopic control until the calyx has been punctured. This is confirmed by aspiration of urine, following which a floppy tip guide wire is advanced across the UPJ.
- Tract dilation then proceeds with either amplatz or balloon dilators up to 30F.

Retrograde tract, Lawson System:
- Retrograde study and placement of a 7.5F deflectable catheter.
- Catheter manoeuvred into a posterior calyx (reduces risk of injury to adjacent structures) with the tip aiming towards the spine.
- Under fluoroscopic guidance a puncture wire is advanced along the ureteric catheter into the calyx and then pushed through the kidney/subcutaneous tissues. A small incision is made in the skin over the wire, which is pulled through.
- The tract can then be dilated up to the desired size.

Contraindications

The main contraindication to percutaneous surgery is a bleeding diathesis; this should be corrected prior to surgery. Relative contraindications to retrograde puncture are obesity, previous renal surgery and dilated collecting systems.

Indications and technique

Percutaneous access to the upper renal tract may be undertaken for either diagnostic or therapeutic purposes. Diagnostic applications include antegrade pyelography, which is mainly used to define the intrarenal collecting system prior to other procedures, and pressure-perfusion studies (the Whitaker test).

The Whitaker test (Whitaker, 1979) involves antegrade perfusion of the renal collecting system at 10ml/min and monitoring the intra renal pressure response. Normal, mild and moderate/severe obstruction are indicated by pressures of <13cm H_2O, 14–22cm H_2O and >22cm H_2O respectively. However, this test has largely been replaced by non-invasive diuretic renograms in more recent years, although it still has a role in more complex cases.

Therapeutic indications can be divided into those for benign and malignant disease:

Benign disease

Nephrostomy drainage
This is often undertaken when retrograde drainage would be inadvisable because of either technically difficult (eg. difficult stones, stricture, tumour) or increased risk to the patient (eg. infected obstructed system). Antegrade drainage is indicated for both intrarenal (eg. obstructed kidney +/- infection, cysts) and perirenal collections (eg. urinoma, perinepheric abscess). The principles for establishing an antegrade nephrostomy have been described above.

Antegrade stenting
This technique is used when a retrograde approach is not possible or has failed. Initially percutaneous guidewire access is obtained via needle puncture. Following this the guidewire, then the stent are directed down the ureter into the bladder under x-ray control.

Treatment of ureteric strictures
Ureteric strictures can be treated endourologically by either balloon dilation (Banner *et al*, 1983) or endoureterotomy (Meretyk *et al*, 1992). Access can be retrograde or antegrade (Mitty *et al*, 1983). Alternatively a combination of both approaches, the rendezvous procedure, can be used (Watson *et al*, 2002). Results for balloon dilation show a 48–88% success rate, with short, non-ischaemic strictures doing better. Endoureterotomy success rates range from 55–85% (Hafez and Wolf, 2003).

Percutaneous Endopyelotomy/Pyelolysis

Since the introduction of endourological management of UPJ obstruction by Ramsay and colleagues in 1984, several variations in technique for performing endopyelotomy have been reported (Badlani *et al*, 1986; Korth *et al*, 1988; Van Cangh *et al*, 1989; Ono *et al*, 1992; Bernardo and Smith, 2000). However the principles of the procedure are common to all and involve gaining percutaneous access via an upper or mid pole calyx. The UPJ is identified and a guide wire passed into the ureter if one has not already been placed retrogradely. A full thickness incision into peripelvic/ureteral fat is made through the stricture and about 1cm below and above it. The incision is made laterally/posterior-laterally to avoid any crossing vessels. A variety of methods for making the incision have been described including cold knife, hooked knife, Bugbee electrode and holmium laser.

Post procedure a JJ stent is sited. The optimum size of stent or duration of stenting is not known, but most auth ors tend to use either an 8F or 14/7F stent for 6–8 weeks. The overall success rate for this procedure is 86% at eight years (Motola *et al*, 1993).

More recently retrograde techniques using either a hot-wire cutting balloon (Chandhoke *et al*, 1993) or ureteroscopic incision (Conlin and Bagley, 1998) have been developed and have equivalent efficacy to the percutaneous technique. In addition, laparoscopic dismembered pyeloplasty is gaining popularity as it appears to have success rates equivalent to open surgery (Jarrett *et al*, 2002). However this is not the end of percutaneous procedures for UPJ obstruction, as will be seen in the next two sections.

Percutaneous endopyeloplasty

This procedure is a modification of percutaneous endopyelotomy. The longitudinal endopyelotomy incision is sutured in a horizontal Heineke-Mikulicz fashion through the solitary percutaneous tract with an in-line suturing device (Gill *et al*, 2002) (*Figure 5.1*) thus achieving a Fenger-plasty type of repair of the UPJ (see *Figure 5.2*). A recent comparison of endopyelotomy, laparoscopic dismembered pyeloplasty and endopyeloplasty with one year follow up showed that resolution of symptoms and improvement in drainage were equivalent in the laparoscopic and endopyeloplasty groups which were both superior to endopyelotomy (Desai *et al*, 2003). However the mean operating time was over two hours shorter for the endopyeloplasty compared to the laparoscopic group. With longer follow up endopyeloplasty may well prove a preferable technique to laparoscopic dismembered pyeloplasty.

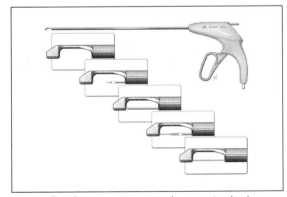

Figure 5.1: Percutaneous nephroscopic dual action suturing device

Percutaneous dismembered pyeloplasty

This technique has recently been developed by Gill and colleagues (Sharp *et al*, 2003) .They have introduced the concept of Percutaneous Intrarenal Reconstructive Surgery (PIRS) and reported a percutaneous Anderson-Hynes type pyeloplasty in a pig model. Their technique involves gaining access to the UPJ via a percutaneous transrenal tract. Carbon dioxide insufflation was employed to visualize the UPJ, which is then dismembered and the proximal ureter dissected and mobilized. The UPJ can then be removed via the tract and a spatulated endopyeloplasty anastomosis created with interrupted sutures using a novel nephroscopic suturing device. Initial results are promising although the technique has yet to be tried in humans.

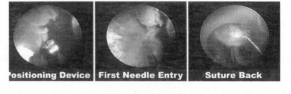

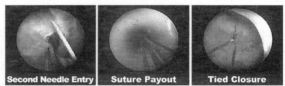

Figure 5.2: Percutaneous intrarenal recontruction

Percutaneous nephrolithotomy (PCNL)

Open surgery, laparoscopic surgery, ureteroscopy, PCNL and ESWL are available modalities to the clinician for treating upper tract stones. The aim of treatment is to render the patient asymptomatic and stone free using the least invasive/morbid method. Taking account of these options the current indications for percutaneous treatment include:

■ Obstruction not caused by the stone (eg. UPJ obstruction or calyceal diverticulum).
■ Stones >20mm diameter (NIH Consensus Conference, 1988).
■ Stones that are not amenable to ESWL or ureteroscopic treatment (eg. renal anomalies, pelvic kidney, and obesity).
■ Infected stones (eg staghorns) (Segura *et al*, 1994).
■ Stones <20mm diameter where the primary treatment modality has failed.
■ Lower pole stones >10mm (Albala *et al*, 2001).

The procedure itself involves fragmenting larger stones either mechanically with a punch, or with ultrasonic, electrohydraulic or laser energy and then removing the fragments with basket/graspers/forceps. During the operation, the collecting system should be irrigated with normal saline as fluid absorption can be significant.

After completion of the procedure a nephrostomy tube is generally placed, although 'tubeless PCNL' is gaining support. Here a JJ stent can be placed prior to removal of the nephrostomy at the end of the procedure (Bellman *et al*, 1997). The advantages of removing the tube are that it reduces postoperative pain, and allows earlier mobilization and return to work. However, if further intervention is required then the tract will have to be re-established.

Success rates can be as high as 99%, but as the stone burden increases, the stone-free rate drops. This can be improved by using multiple percutaneous tracts or repeating the surgery within forty-eight hours of the initial procedure (once bleeding has settled and vision improved). In addition percutaneous interventions can be combined with ESWL and ureteroscopic methods to improve clearance.

Malignant disease

Percutaneous treatment of upper tract (TCC)

In patients with bilateral tumours, solitary kidneys or severe co-morbidities endoscopic resection of upper tract TCC is an option that allows treatment of the tumour with renal preservation. This was first described by Tomera and colleagues (Tomera *et al*, 1982). The procedure involves establishing a percutaneous tract and using either electrocautery or laser energy for resection and hemostasis. Deep biopsies of the tumour bed can also be taken allowing stage to be established. Generally a nephrostomy tube is left in place that allows a second-look nephroscopy at four to fourteen days; this ensures that all tumour has been removed. If adjuvant topical therapy is required, the nephrostomy tube can be exchanged for an 8F tube that can be left for the duration of treatment.

Outcome can be predicted by tumour grade: the recurrence rates for grade one, two and three tumours are 18%, 33% and 50% respectively (Jarrett *et al*, 1995). With thirteen years of follow-up it has been shown that there is no difference in overall survival when comparing percutaneous resection with nephroureterectomy (Lee *et al*, 1999).

Percutaneous resection has two main advantages over ureteroscopic resection: firstly, with larger tumour burdens clearance is more easily facilitated and secondly, it can stage tumours in addition to grading them. Although there is a possibility of tract seeding, the largest series have not reported any cases of this (Jarrett *et al*, 1995; Patel *et al*, 1996; Clark *et al*, 1999) despite several case reports in the literature (Tomera *et al*, 1982; Slywotzky and Maya, 1994; Huang *et al*, 1995). To obviate this possibility an iridium wire combined with intrarenal chemotherapy seems to have some theoretical advantages.

In summary, the literature generally agrees that it is reasonable to manage grade one upper tract TCC percutaneously, provided that the patient is willing to have lifelong endoscopic follow-up. Grade three disease should generally be managed with nephroureterectomy. There is currently no consensus on the management of grade two disease with a normal contralateral kidney. In addition success depends on both stage and grade of the tumour: the lower the grade of TCC the more favourable the outcome.

Percutaneous treatment of renal cell carcinoma

The widespread use of abdominal imaging with US, CT and MRI has led to an increase in the number of incidentally detected renal masses, often at a much earlier stage (Pantuck *et al*, 2000). As a result nephron-sparing surgery either open or laparoscopic has become more popular for treating these tumours. For patients who are not candidates for or have refused open/laparoscopic surgery percutaneous radiofrequency (Zagoria, 2003) or cryoablation (Uchida *et al*, 1995) techniques are an option. With both techniques the energy sources are positioned in the lesion percutaneously under CT guidance. Uchida's group only performed the cryoablation in two patients with metastatic disease, but both patients had significant shrinkage of the lesion on follow-up CT scans. Radio frequency ablation has been more widely used. Results with follow-up up to a year show that no growth or residual enhancements are present in up to 85% of patients (Su *et al*, 2003). Although early results are encouraging, long-term follow-up is necessary to establish the precise role in this patient population.

Complications of percutaneous access

Percutaneous surgery has significantly decreased the morbidity of equivalent open surgical procedures (Farrell and Hicks, 1997). Attempts to further reduce the complications of percutaneous procedures have been advanced by the introduction of the 'mini-perc', which is reported to cause less hemorrhage and postoperative pain (Jackman *et al*, 1998). The complications that arise from percutaneous surgery are related to the tract and the procedure performed. These include:

Haemorrhage

This can occur acutely from damage to intrarenal (usually calyceal neck vessels) or perinepheric vessels and is best managed by tamponade eg. with a large nephrostomy tube. Rarely angiography and embolization or open surgery may be required (Kessaris *et al*, 1995). Late bleeding after nephrostomy removal is unusual. A-V fistula formation is a rare late complication which can be managed by embolization.

Injuries to the collecting system

Small perforations can occur in around 7% of PCNL procedures (Lee *et al*, 1987). This usually resolves with nephrostomy drainage. Larger perforations of the renal pelvis are uncommon and mostly heal with antegrade stent placement and nephrostomy drainage. Larger perforations that do not heal may require open surgical repair, but occur in <1% of cases (Lee *et al*, 1987).

Injury to adjacent structures

The pleura/lung, liver, spleen, colon and duodenum can all sustain injury during percutaneous procedures. The lung and pleura are at greatest risk, especially with a supracostal tract. Pneumothorax has been reported in 0–4% and pleural effusion in 0–8% with a supracostal approach (Picus *et al*, 1986; Forsyth and Fuchs, 1987). A postoperative chest x-ray should be taken after supracostal procedures, a small pneumothorax or effusion can be left or aspirated, larger clinically significant injuries may require a chest drain. Among the other organs injured the colon is most common and occurs in <1% of cases (Lee *et al*, 1987). If the perforation is retroperitoneal then these injuries can be managed by pulling the nephrostomy tube back into the colon, placing a retrograde JJ stent and treating with antibiotics. Open surgical management is only required if this conservative management fails or there are signs of peritonitis/sepsis.

Other complications

These include loss of nephrostomy tract, sepsis, fluid overload, retained fragments, stricture, leakage from around the nephrostomy tube and late hypertension.

Conclusions

The development of percutaneous surgery has allowed many conditions that previously required major open surgery to be treated endoscopically, with considerable reductions in morbidity, mortality and cost. It is now one of the main minimally invasive treatment options for large stone burdens, UPJ obstruction, strictures and upper tract lesions. The future of percutaneous surgery looks promising, with applications of this technique continuing to grow with improvements in technology and reduction in morbidity.

> ## Key points for *Chapter 5*
>
> - Bleeding diathesis is the major contraindication to percutaneous surgery; normal clotting studies must be established prior to the procedure.
> - Access is most commonly obtained with the antegrade approach.
> - The ideal site for puncture is through a posterior calyx, as this reduces the likelihood of vascular injury.
> - A retrograde approach may be preferred for hypermobile or malrotated kidneys.
> - PCNL is indicated for upper tract calculi >20mm diameter, or lower pole calculi >10mm. Other indications include obstruction not caused by the stone, failure or unsuitability of other treatment modalities and infected stones.
> - Multiple percutaneous treatment sessions and/or combination with other modalities improves clearance rates for high stone burdens.
> - Percutaneous management of grade one upper tract TCC with lifelong endoscopic follow up allows improved histological staging and clearance of large tumour burden over ureteroscopic methods. The tract also allows chemo and immonotherapy to be applied.
> - Patients with renal cell carcinoma who are unsuitable for surgery may be offered percutaneous radiofrequency or cryoablation techniques. The long term results of these are awaited.
> - Complications include: injury to the collecting system, injury to surrounding structures, sepsis, loss of the tract, fluid overload, retained fragments, stricture, leakage from around the nephrostomy tube and late hypertension.

References

Albala DM, Assimos DG *et al* (2001) Lower pole I: a prospective randomized trial of extracorporeal shock wave lithotripsy and percutaneous nephrostolithotomy for lower pole nephrolithiasis-initial results. *J Urol* **166(6):** 2072–80

Badlani G, Eshghi M *et al* (1986) Percutaneous surgery for ureteropelvic junction obstruction (endopyelotomy). Technique and early results. *J Urol* **135:** 26

Banner MP, Pollack HM *et al* (1983) Catheter dilatation of benign ureteral strictures. *Radiology* **147:** 427–33

Bellman GC, Davidoff R *et al* (1997) Tubeless percutaneous renal surgery. *J Urol* **157(5):** 1578–82

Bernardo NO, Smith AD (2000) Percutaneous endopyelotomy. *Urology* **56(2):** 322–7

Chandhoke PS, Clayman RV *et al* (1993) Endopyelotomy and endoureterotomy with the Acucise ureteral cutting balloon device: Preliminary experience. *J Endourol* **7:** 45

Clark PC, Streem SB *et al* (1999) 13 year experience with percutaneous management of upper tract transitional cell carcinoma. *J Urol* **161:** 772–75

Conlin MJ, Bagley DH (1998) Ureteroscopic endopyelotomy at a single setting. *J Urol* **159:** 727

Desai M, Gill I *et al* (2003) Percutaneous endopyeloplasty. Intermediate term results and comparison with endopyelotomy and laparoscopic pyeloplasty. *J Endourol* **17(Suppl.1):** MP27.12

Farrell TA, Hicks ME (1997) A review of radiologically guided percutaneous nephrostomies in 303 patients. *J Vasc Intervent Radiol* **8(5):** 769–74

Fernstrom I, Johansson B (1976) Percutaneous pyelolithotomy. A new extraction technique. *Scand J Urol Nephrol* **10(3):** 257–9

Forsyth MJ, Fuchs EE (1987) The supracostal approach for percutaneous nephrostolithotomy. *J Urol* **137:** 197

Gill IS, Desai MM *et al* (2002) Percutaneous endopyeloplasty: Description of a new technique. *J Urol* **168:** 2097–2102

Hafez KS and Wolf JS (2003) Update on minimally invasive management of ureteral strictures. *J Endourol* **17(7):** 453–64

Hosking DH (1996) Retrograde access. In Smith AD, Badlani GH, Kavoussi LR, *et al* (eds): *Smith's Textbook of Endourology*. Quality Medical, St Louis 211

Huang A, Low RK *et al* (1995) Nephrostomy tract tumor seeding following percutaneous manipulation of a ureteral carcinoma. *J Urol* **153:** 1041–42

Jackman SV, Docimo SG *et al* (1998) The 'mini-perc' technique: A less invasive alternative to percutaneous nephrolithotomy. *World J Urol* **16:** 371

Jarrett TW, Chan DY *et al* (2002) Laparoscopic pyeloplasty: the first 100 cases. *J Urol* **167(3):** 1253–6

Jarrett TW, Sweetser PM *et al* (1995) Percutaneous management of transitional cell carcinoma of the renal collecting system: 9-year experience. *J Urol* **154:** 1629–35

Kessaris DN, Bellman GC *et al* (1995) Management of hemorrhage after percutaneous renal surgery. *J Urol* **153:** 604

Korth K, Kuenkel M *et al* (1988) Percutaneous pyeloplasty. *Urology* **31:** 503

Lee BR, Jabbour ME *et al* (1999) 13-year survival comparison of percutaneous and open nephroureterectomy approaches for management of transitional cell carcinoma of renal collecting system: equivalent outcomes. *J Endourol* **13(4):** 289–94

Lee WJ, Smith AD *et al* (1987) Complications of percutaneous nephrolithotomy. *AJR Am J Roentgenol* **148(1):** 177–80

LeRoy AJ (1996) Percutaneous access. In Smith AD, Badlani GH, Kavoussi LR, *et al* (eds): *Smith's Textbook of Endourology*. Quality Medical, St Louis 199

Meretyk S, Albala DM *et al* (1992) Endoureterotomy for treatment of ureteral strictures. *J Urol* **147(6):** 1502–6

Mitty HA, Train JS *et al* (1983) Antegrade ureteral stenting in the management of fistulas, strictures, and calculi. *Radiology* **149:** 433

Motola JA, Badlani GH *et al* (1993) Results of 212 consecutive endopyelotomies: an 8-year followup. *J Urol* **149(3):** 453–6

NIH Consensus Conference, 1988

Ono Y, Ohshima S *et al* (1992) Endopyeloureterotomy via a transpelvic extraureteral approach. *J Urol* **147:** 352

Pantuck AJ, Zisman A *et al* (2000) Incidental renal tumors. *Urology* **56(2):** 190–6

Patel A, Soonawalla P *et al* (1996) Long-term outcome after percutaneous treatment of transitional cell carcinoma of the renal pelvis. *J Urol* **155:** 868–74

Picus D, Weyman PJ *et al* (1986) Intercostal-space nephrostomy for percutaneous stone removal. *Am J Roentgenol* **147:** 393

Ramsay JWA, Miller RA *et al* (1984) Percutaneous pyelolysis: Indications, complications and results. *Br J Urol* **56:** 586

Segura JW, Preminger GM *et al* (1994) Nephrolithiasis clinical guidelines panel summary report on the management of staghorn calculi. *J Urol* **151:** 1648–51

Sharp DS, Desai M *et al* (2003) Dismembered percutaneous endopyeloplasty: a new procedure. *J Endourol* **17(Suppl.1):** MP06.09

Slywotzky C, Maya M (1994) Needle tract seeding of transitional cell carcinoma following fine-needle aspiration of a renal mass. *Abdom Imaging* **19:** 174–76

Su LM, Jarrett TW *et al* (2003) Percutaneous computed tomography-guided radiofrequency ablation of renal masses in high surgical risk patients: preliminary results. *Urology* **61(4 Suppl 1):** 26–33

Tomera KM, Leary FJ *et al* (1982) Pyeloscopy in urothelial tumors. *J Urol* **127:** 1088–89

Uchida M, Imaide Y *et al* (1995) Percutaneous cryosurgery for renal tumours. *Br J Urol* **75(2):** 132–6

Van Cangh PJ, Jorion JL *et al* (1989) Endoureteropyelotomy: Percutaneous treatment of ureteropelvic junction obstruction. *J Urol* **141:** 1317

Watson JM, Dawkins GPC *et al* (2002) The rendezvous procedure to cross complicated ureteric strictures. *BJU Int* **89(3):** 317–19

Whitaker RH (1979) An evaluation of 170 diagnostic pressure flow studies of the upper urinary tract. *J Urol* **121(5):** 602–4

Zagoria RJ (2003) Percutaneous image-guided radiofrequency ablation of renal malignancies. *Radiol Clin North Am* **41(5):** 1067–75

CHAPTER 6

Ureteroscopy

R Madeb, J Boczko, E Erturk

Although ureteroscopes were initially developed to treat lower ureteral stones, modern technological advancement has led to their ever expanding roles in the field of urology. Ureteroscopes are currently used in the diagnosis and treatment of many upper urinary tract diseases such as UPJ obstruction, ureteral strictures and upper tract urothelial malignancy. In this chapter, we describe the two main types of ureteroscopes and the techniques required for their use; the indications for use, possible complications, controversies with current day ureteroscopy, and the role of virtual ureteroscopy are also discussed.

Introduction

Ureteroscopes were initially developed to gain access to the lower ureter in order to remove distal ureteral stones under visual guidance. Currently, most stones, especially those in the kidney and upper collecting system are managed with minimally invasive techniques including shockwave lithotripsy and/or ureteroscopy. With improvement in technology, the urologist can now safely visualize the entire urinary tract, and perform both diagnostic and therapeutic procedures with minimal morbidity.

Instrumentation

Since their introduction, ureteroscopes have undergone significant modifications (Basillote *et al*, 2004; Johnston *et al*, 2004). The first-generation ureteroscopes were larger in diameter compared to current-day scopes and were very similar to rigid cystoscopes. Several changes were made to the original ureteroscope that allowed it to be more easily inserted into the ureteral orifices while maintaining its dual ability to give clear visual field and working channels (Bagley *et al*, 1983; Basillote *et al*, 2004). The first advancement was the reduction of scope diameter from 11–13Fr to 6–9Fr. These smaller diameter scopes however, posed a new challenge. They were prone to bending which, as in the classic rod lens system, led to breakage of the lens and loss of optimal visualization. To make the ureteroscope more functional, the metal casing on the thinner scopes was modified to allow extreme bending without breakage. Subsequently, fiber optic lenses were introduced, leading to our current day semi-rigid ureteroscope (*Figure 6.1*). These changes allowed the ureteroscopes to retain their optic power while being bent and yet, stay thin and somewhat flexible (Bagley *et al* 1983; Abdel-Razzak and Bagley, 1992). Another important modification was the separation of the working port from the irrigation channel. This enabled continuous irrigation for visualization with the simultaneous ability of inserting instruments through the working element. Currently, the working ports of semi-rigid ureteroscopes are 3Fr and can accept a variety of different endoscopic instruments.

With the development of fiber optic technology, we now have completely flexible cystoscopes and ureteroscopes with active deflection, (*Figure 6.2*) allowing the manipulation required to pass these instruments into the upper urinary tract (Bagley *et al* 1983; Abdel-Razzak and Bagley, 1992; Afane *et al*, 2000). The most remote locations of the renal collecting system can now be easily reached without significant trauma, opening a whole range of minimally invasive diagnostic and therapeutic options (Basillote *et al*, 2004).

Technique

Semi-rigid ureteroscopy is performed under direct vision and fluoroscopic guidance. With the patient in the standard lithotomy position, cystoscopy is performed to scan the normal anatomical landmarks and assess for any bladder pathology. Once the ureteral orifice is identified, a floppy guide wire is passed up the ureter into the collecting system of the kidney. The ureteroscope is then advanced up the lower urinary tract, following the wire or over a second wire if needed. A wire should be kept in place as a safety guide wire throughout the procedure, to allow access to the collecting system even in the face of ureteral trauma or edema. If direct passage of the scope through the ureteral orifice is not possible, secondary to narrowing or stricture, the distal ureter may be dilated with a graduated 10Fr ureteral dilator or a 16–22Fr ureteral balloon dilator. In the majority of cases, the ureter below the iliac vessels can be easily reached with a semi-rigid scope. However, access to the ureteral segment above the iliac vessels can be difficult with a semi-rigid

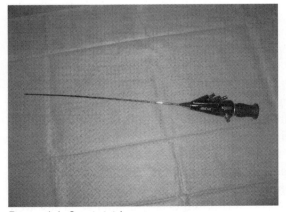

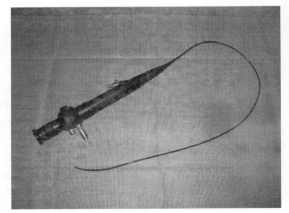

Figure 6.1: Semi-rigid ureteroscope   *Figure 6.2: Flexible ureteroscope*

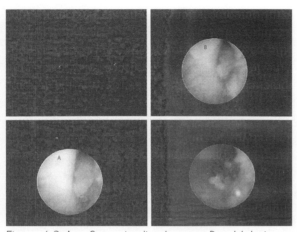

Figure 6.3: A – Stone in distal ureter. B – Holmium laser being focused on stone. C – Small stone fragments following laser lithotripsy

scope due to its anatomical curvature. A flexible ureteroscope is generally recommended for proximal ureteral access in order to avoid injury.

While flexible ureteroscopy allows unrestricted motion through the curves of the ureter, the inherent flexibility of the instrument can make entrance into the ureteral orifice difficult. Dilation of the ureteral orifice, or distal ureter may therefore be necessary. For specific cases requiring multiple entries into the ureter, it is often necessary to use a ureteral access sheath. This allows the flexible ureteroscope to be inserted and removed multiple times as needed without injury to the ureter. These access sheaths are available in different diameters and lengths, and usually have a hydrophilic coating enabling adherence to the ureteral wall. These sheaths optimize visualization through the ability to irrigate faster.

Ureteroscopic treatment of ureteral stones

Semi-rigid ureteroscopes are generally used to treat stones in the distal ureter, while flexible ureteroscopes are used for stones located proximally, or in the kidney (Lingeman *et al*, 1986; Grocela and Dretler, 1997). Ureteral stones can be either directly removed or pulverized with a variety of intracorporeal lithotripters (Zheng and Denstedt, 2000). Ureteral stones less than 5mm can be retrieved with ureteroscopic baskets or grasping forceps. It is crucial during stone extraction that both the ureteral wall and stone be continuously monitored endoscopically, and fluoroscopically to avoid avulsion of the ureter. For stones located in the upper urinary tract, including the kidney, insertion of a ureteral access sheath as discussed above, may facilitate stone removal. The working channel of flexible ureteroscopes varies between 3 and 3.6Fr. Since there are no separate irrigation ports adequate visualization can be compromised with the passage of instruments. A pressurized irrigation system is often required to maintain adequate flow. It is also important that instruments introduced through the ureteroscope be flexible to avoid compromising the scope's working element. Recent developments with nitinol technology have led to durable and malleable baskets and forceps. These instruments have allowed procedures previously impossible to be performed with ease in the upper urinary tract and renal pelvis.

Ureteroscopic management of UPJ obstruction

Endoscopic management of UPJ obstruction has become common during the last decade. This procedure relies on a full thickness incision of the ureteral narrowing and subsequent stenting for secondary healing (Gerber *et al*, 2000). Early attempts to perform this procedure with semi-rigid ureteroscopes and electrocautery units achieved marginal success rates and many complications. The development of flexible ureteroscopes and lasers allows complete access to the upper urinary tract and greatly improves success rates while decreasing complication rates (Osther *et al*, 1998; Tawfiek *et al*, 1998; Gerber *et al*, 2000). Prior to making an incision with a 200-micron holmium laser fiber under direct vision, a safety guide wire is inserted into the kidney that can be used for passage of a ureteral stent. The ureter is then cut full thickness, usually anterolaterally (*Figure 6.4*). Subsequently, the ureter is stented with a double pigtail stent

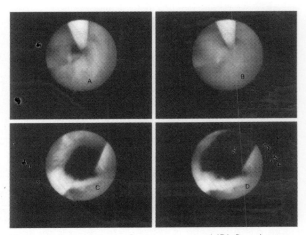

Figure 6.4: A – View of narrowing at UPJ. B – Laser beam focused in preparation for ureterolysis. C – Opening in previously obstructed UPJ beginning to open. D – Final widely opened UPJ

for at least three to four weeks to permit ureteral healing and to minimize recurrent narrowing. Before performing this procedure, it is advisable to image the kidney with a CT scan to rule out aberrant renal vessels that may be the cause of the narrowing. If such vessels are present, endoscopic treatment is contraindicated due to risk of vessel injury. The advantage of this procedure is reduced morbidity compared to percutaneous and antegrade endopyelotomy (Osther *et al*, 1998; Tawfiek *et al*, 1998; Gerber *et al*, 2000). Risks of hemorrhage and injury to the kidney are significantly reduced. The procedure can be performed in an outpatient setting and does not require percutaneous access. The long-term results have been relatively successful compared to both antegrade endopyelotomy and open pyeloplasty (Desai *et al*, 2004). Although success rates are lower, secondary UPJ obstruction has also been successfully treated with this method.

Ureteroscopic management of ureteral strictures

Ureteral strictures can be managed with ureteroscopes in a retrograde fashion (Kim and Gerber, 2000). Depending on their etiology and length, ureteral strictures will respond variably to this form of intervention. Typically, short and idiopathic strictures have the best outcomes. Ischemic and traumatic strictures are typically resistant to any form of endoscopic intervention. Surgical technique is similar to that used in the treatment of a UPJ obstruction. A full thickness ureteral incision is made after a guide wire passed into the kidney. Holmium laser is commonly used for this procedure. Depending upon the location of the stricture, either the flexible or semi-rigid ureteroscope can be utilized. Subsequently, the ureter is stented for several weeks. The older, more conventional open procedure in treating ureteral strictures, not only carries serious potential risks, but also might not be possible due to co-morbid medical conditions. These instances include renal transplant ureteral strictures, uretero-enteric fistula strictures, secondary UPJ obstruction, post ureteroscopy or ureteral surgery strictures and radiation strictures (Kim and Gerber, 2000).

Ureteroscopic management of urothelial malignancies

The development of modern ureteroscopes has greatly impacted on the treatment and diagnosis of ureteral tumors (Bagley *et al*, 1987; Huffman, 1989). These lesions can now be directly seen and biopsied for accurate pathologic diagnosis (Abdel-Razzak *et al*, 1994). This in turn has resulted in successful management of low-grade, non-invasive tumors with minimally invasive techniques, thus sparing the need for nephrectomy or nephroureterectomy. This treatment option is especially useful in patients who are poor candidates for surgery, or those with compromised renal function or a solitary kidney. Furthermore, after definitive endoscopic surgery, regular surveillance can be easily performed with minimal morbidity to the patient. Prior to the introduction of lasers, tissue ablation required electrocautery units. These probes generally had large diameters and therefore were limited to the distal ureter. Laser fibers, as small as 200 microns, are easily inserted through smaller, flexible ureteroscopes and exhibit superior tissue destruction and hemostasis. Technically, the procedure is performed in a similar fashion to that used in ureteroscopy for stone disease. It is crucial to maintain both adequate visualization and have a safety wire throughout the procedure. Initially, using a small biopsy forceps, tissue is obtained to confirm the pathology. Subsequently the visible tumor is ablated. The upper ureter and the pelvocalyceal system are best visualized with flexible ureteroscopes, thereby only allowing small, flexible instruments to be used. Indications for a retrograde approach in the management of urothelial malignancies depend upon location, size, and malignant potential of the lesion. It is important to recognize the limitations with this approach when dealing with malignant lesions in the upper collecting system, as high-grade, invasive urothelial tumors can spread rapidly and opportunities to cure with radical surgery may be quickly lost.

Complications

With refinement of ureteroscopic techniques and instrumentation, complication rates have significantly decreased (Huffman, 1989; Johnson and Pearle, 2004). The primary complication, especially with semi-rigid ureteroscopes, is ureteral perforation (Huffman, 1989; Johnson and Pearle, 2004). Such perforations are usually minor and often can be conservatively treated with ureteral stenting. Small perforations may result from stone fragmentation either by laser or EHL (Electrohydraulic Lithotripsy) probes. Larger perforations may result from forceful introduction of ureteroscopes into the ureter. Significant ureteral tear and avulsion is generally the result of aggressive stone extraction and is extremely rare. This complication should be recognized early. Ureteral reimplantation may be necessary to avoid significant morbidity. Occasionally a ureteral stone can migrate into the retroperitoneum. In this situation, the stone can be left without further intervention. Infected and impacted stones in the ureteral wall can lead to ureteral scarring and ultimately stricture. Significant bleeding during ureteroscopy is extremely rare and is usually the result of inadvertent incision of aberrant blood vessels during treatment of UPJ obstruction or stricture disease. This can be largely avoided with preoperative radiographic imaging. Bleeding during tumor ablation is generally self-limiting and rarely requires aggressive management. Long-term complications of ureteroscopy are limited to ureteral strictures, which have decreased to approximately 1%. Overall complication rates following ureteroscopy varies between two and 6% (Huffman, 1989; Johnson and Pearle, 2004).

Controversies in ureteroscopy

Choosing the Right Procedure: How Does Location Affect Treatment Options?

Multiple factors such as stone size, location, composition, previous stone history, body habitus, patient and surgeon preference, and previous surgical treatments help guide the decision in choosing the best method for treatment of ureteral stones (Segura *et al*, 1997). Guidelines are being established, however, they do not support the superiority of one treatment option over another. Thus, selecting the most optimal treatment for proximal and distal ureteral stones remains controversial.

Distal ureteral stones

The treatment for distal ureteral stones remains one of the most heavily debated subjects in urology. The debate stems from the fact that access to the distal ureter in the twenty-first century is easily accomplished with current day semi-rigid ureteroscopes. This allows for direct visualization and pulverization of the stone, leading to high stone free rates. In contrast, proponents of Shock Wave Lithotripsy (SWL) feel that ureteroscopy is invasive and excellent stone-free rates can be accomplished with shock wave lithotripsy. This issue has been evaluated in many retrospective studies comparing ureteroscopy to Shock Wave Lithotripsy (SWL). Most major studies agree that success rates are generally higher with ureteroscopy than with SWL treatments (Erturk and Herrman, 1993; Anderson *et al*, 1994; Peschel *et al*, 1999). Despite these data, some groups still recommend SWL as first-line therapy (Erturk and Herrman, 1993; Anderson *et al*, 1994; Peschel *et al*, 1999). Prospective randomized trials have also started to tackle this dilemma. The first study performed by Peschel and colleagues (Peschel *et al*, 1999) reported a complete ureteroscopic stone-free rate (forty patients) and 90% SWL stone-free rate on a Dornier MFL5000 lithotripter (forty patients). For stones of <5 mm or >5 mm in diameter, the SWL stone-free rates were 95% and 85%, respectively. The procedure was faster in the ureteroscopy arm and no complications were seen in either group. Of interest, 100% of the patients were satisfied with ureteroscopy compared to just 85% after SWL. The study concluded that ureteroscopic stone extraction should be recommended as first-line therapy for distal stones. Conversely, Pearle *et al* (Pearle *et al*, 2001) prospectively randomized thirty-two patients with distal stones (diameter <1.5 cm) to ureteroscopy or SWL on a HM3 lithotripter. Both treatments cleared the stones completely. SWL was associated with fewer perioperative complications, less postoperative discomfort, and greater overall patient satisfaction, causing the group to conclude that SWL with a HM3 lithotripter should be used as first-line treatment for distal stones.

We think that ideally, current technical and practical issues make ureteroscopy the favored treatment for distal stones. On a practical basis, the lower ureter can be accessed with a semi-rigid or flexible instrument in nearly 100% of the cases. Compared with SWL, ureteroscopy is associated with a higher stone-free rate and requires fewer secondary interventions. Most importantly, patients typically can have a successful outcome after just one surgical procedure. However, access to an operating room might be more challenging than with an SWL suite. Therefore, despite ureteroscopy having higher stone-free rates, it might be quicker and more cost-efficient to treat patients with SWL therapy at some centers.

Proximal ureteral stones

Historically, management of proximal ureteral stones has been primarily with SWL. Since the advent of fiber optics in endourology and ureteroscopy, proximal ureteral stones have been increasingly treated with the flexible ureteroscope. Initially, ureteroscope design did not particularly facilitate stone treatment in the proximal ureter (see section above). This, in conjunction with poor ureteroscopic success rates for proximal ureteral stones, (Segura *et al*, 1997) and the ease of use of the newer SWL machines had led urologists to shy away from retrograde access and treatment of proximal ureteral stones. In addition, ureteroscopy of the upper collecting system was technically more challenging than SWL, making SWL the modality of choice for upper collecting system stones. Concurrent with the development of flexible ureteroscopes, Ho:YAG laser and potentially with the replacement of the Dornier HM3 lithotripter with second and third-generation machines, an increased use in ureteroscopic treatment of proximal ureteral stones has been documented.

Contemporary reports show comparable success rates for ureteroscopic treatment of proximal ureteral stones. Between 1998 and 2003, several SWL series published a 75% overall stone free-rate using second- or third-generation lithotriptors (Yip *et al*, 1998; Matsuoka *et al*, 1999). The re-treatment rate was 30% among patients in these reports with a 9.4% ancillary procedure rate. Conversely, ureteroscopy series for proximal ureteral stones published between 1995 and 2003, revealed an 82% stone rate with a 10% second-procedure rate (Yip *et al*, 1998; Matsuoka *et al*, 1999). The overall ureteroscopy complication rate decreased to 6.6% when treating proximal ureteral stones.

Although multiple studies have shown superiority for ureteroscopic treatment of proximal stones, several issues need to be addressed before deeming ureteroscopy the optimal choice for management of proximal ureteral stone disease. First, unlike distal ureteral stone management, ureteroscopy of the upper collecting system is technically more challenging than SWL and distal ureteroscopy. Moreover, there are many more other pathologies that can preclude upper collecting system ureteroscopy including anatomical variations, pyelonephritis, strictures, and urinary diversion. At our institution, despite an increase in the numbers of proximal ureteral stones treated with ureteroscopy, we still favor SWL as first-line therapy for most proximal ureteral stones.

To sheath or not to sheath?

Another dilemma that has developed among endourologists involves the use of access sheaths during ureteroscopy. Access sheaths were initially introduced to aid difficult access to the ureter (Kourambas *et al*, 2001; Delvecchio *et al*, 2003). Their use has since broadened to include dilating ureters and possibly facilitating ureteroscope placement. Moreover, when performing flexible ureteroscopy of the upper collecting system, multiple insertions and removals of the ureteroscope can be performed without re-manipulation or (iatrogenic) trauma to the ureter. There have been a handful of studies that address this controversy. Kourambas *et al* (Kourambas *et al*, 2001) compared patients undergoing ureteroscopy with or without a ureter access sheath. They reported a greater incidence of postoperative symptoms for patients who required balloon ureteral *vs*. access sheath dilatation alone. More importantly, the use of a ureteral access sheath decreased the operative time and costs among the study patients. A criticism in the use of access sheaths is the possible complications of stricture that may result from large diameter tubes (10–16F) in the ureter. Although it is too early to have sufficient long term data, short-term follow-up, has shown that newer generation access sheaths are safe and effective with a 1.4% incidence of strictures (Kourambas *et al*, 2001; Delvecchio *et al*, 2003). In our experience, ureteral access sheaths have also facilitated intrarenal and proximal ureteroscopy and are selectively used for the treatment of difficult proximal ureteral calculi. Clearly, additional reports on the efficacy of access sheaths and long-term complication rates are warranted before this question can be answered.

To stent or not to stent?

Stents have routinely been placed after ureteroscopic procedures to facilitate stone clearance and avoid complications such as flank pain secondary to ureteral edema. Although the placement of a ureteral stent may be helpful, the presence of a ureteral stent is associated with significant morbidity and a decrease in quality of life. Stents may cause urinary symptoms (such as urgency, frequency and dysuria) and suprapubic pain. Multiple studies with different levels of evidence including retrospective, prospective non-randomized, and prospective randomized studies have found uncomplicated ureteroscopy to be safe with no indwelling ureteral stent (Netto *et al*, 2001; Hollenbeck *et al*, 2003; Joshi *et al*, 2003). One of the most important factors to remember while interpreting these studies is that selection criteria for stent-less ureteroscopy remains an important consideration. Only when strict inclusion criteria are used, such as, inclusion of small distal stones that could be adequately fragmented or removed with no ureteral dilatation or significant ureteral trauma, (Netto *et al*, 2001; Hollenbeck *et al*, 2003; Joshi *et al*, 2003) have the studies shown stent-less ureteroscopy to be effective. For patients meeting these types of inclusion criteria, many patient-related benefits were realized, including decreased postoperative pain, urinary symptoms, operative time and procedural costs (Netto *et al*, 2001; Hollenbeck *et al*, 2003; Joshi *et al*, 2003). Other studies using less stringent inclusion criteria (no limitations on stone burden, ureteral location, degree of obstruction), reported similar patient-related benefits for ureteral stones treated with uncomplicated ureteroscopy. Overall, we feel that stent-less ureteroscopy can be performed in a highly select group of patients with stones treated in the distal ureter. Clearly, routine stenting for all patients after ureteroscopy is unnecessary and ultimately lies in the judgment of the endoscopist.

A look to the future: Virtual ureteroscopy

The incorporation of ureteroscopy and other minimally invasive procedures in endourology has greatly changed the landscape of urology. With these advancements, comes the burden of acquiring the skills needed to successfully perform these procedures. Surgical simulation has emerged in the last decade as a potential tool for aiding acquisition of technical skills, including anesthesia protocols, trauma management, cardiac catheterization and laparoscopy. Recently, advances in virtual reality simulation offer a practical tool for urologists to practice various endourologic procedures ranging from basic to complex in an inanimate but dynamic lifelike environment without risk to patients. Moreover, since endourologic procedures, such as ureteroscopy, requires little in the way of tactile feedback, virtual cystoscopy and ureteroscopy are rapidly gaining acceptance. Immersion Medical, Gaithersburg, Maryland was the first company to build a virtual ureteroscopy simulator.

This simulator allowed urologists to explore the ureter and kidney for pathologic processes, specifically, stones and tumors, however, was limited in capacity due to poor 3-D visualization and anatomic representations. Recent advances in computing power, 3-D software, virtual reality graphics, and physical modeling techniques have resulted in a new endoscopic simulator (URO Mentor system, Symbionix, Tel Aviv, Israel). This commercially available, virtual reality modular endoscopic simulator provides virtual cystoscopy and ureteroscopy procedures using either rigid or flexible endoscopes. Real-time fluoroscopy with simulation of C-arm control and viewing of fluoroscopic images of injected contrast can also be combined with endoscopic procedures. Various endourologic procedures can be simulated realistically, including cystoscopy, retrograde pyelography, insertion of a guidewire, ureteral stenting, ureteroscopy, stone fragmentation, and fragment removal using various tools. In addition, simulated tumor resection and treatment of stricture and obstruction can be reproduced (Michel *et al*, 2002). This has been validated in recent studies which demonstrate that virtual simulators resulted in rapid acquisition of ureteroscopic skills by urologic trainees (Watterson *et al*, 2002). It seems very likely that surgical simulators will play a role in training in the future, and will ultimately have a diagnostic role as 3-D software and virtual reality graphics become more advanced.

Conclusions

The development of newer ureteroscopes has allowed the endourologist to perform a greater number of procedures with decreased morbidity. The semi-rigid scope is more suitable in the distal ureter, while the flexible ureteroscope can be used to access the entire ureter and kidney. In the search for decreased invasiveness, the use of the ureteroscope may persist as it disappears in others. In the areas of stone disease, the advent of ureteroscopes can allow complete stone evacuation at once, which was previously possible only with open surgery. Despite being less morbid, they remain fairly invasive when compared with other established modalities such as shock wave lithotripsy, perpetuating controversies regarding which technology is most suitable in one situation versus another. In the area of diagnostic ureteroscopy, the limitations and invasiveness of available ureteroscopes may soon lead to their replacement with virtual endoscopic techniques where more accurate information may be obtained without physically entering the urinary tract.

Key points for *Chapter 6*

- Ureteroscopes have undergone modifications since their original development that make them more effective in accessing and treating upper urinary tract disease.

- There are specific techniques for using both semi-rigid and flexible ureteroscopes which, when applied, allow for access to the collecting system in a variety of situations.

- The indications for using either a flexible or a semi-rigid ureteroscope may differ according to location of the lesion or stone, or the pathology being managed.

- The most common application of ureteroscopes is in the treatment and removal of ureteral stones. Treatment can be performed throughout the urinary tract.

- Ureteroscopes can be used to treat UPJ obstruction endoscopically, in a minimally invasive manner.

- Ureteroscopes can be used to treat ureteral strictures endoscopically, and to treat urothelial malignancy in the upper urinary tract. .

- The limitations of treating upper tract urothelial malignancy endoscopically must be understood prior to initiating such therapy as high-grade tumors can progress rapidly and require more invasive management.

- Complications, although rare, do occur with the use of ureteroscopes and the proper management of such complications must be understood.

- There are multiple areas of controversy with current day (2005) ureteroscopy including optimal treatment of stones by location, the need for routine stenting after ureteroscopy, the need to use ureteral access sheath.

- The most exciting field in ureteroscopy is the development of virtual simulators for training urologic surgeons. It seems very likely that surgical simulators will play a role in training in the future, and will ultimately have a diagnostic role as 3-D software and virtual reality graphics become more advanced.

References

Abdel-Razzak OM, Bagley DH (1992) Clinical experience with flexible ureteropyeloscopy. *J Urol* **148(6):** 1788–92

Abdel-Razzak OM, Ehya H *et al* (1994) Ureteroscopic biopsy in the upper urinary tract. *Urology* **44(3):** 451–7

Afane JS, Olweny EO *et al* (2000) Flexible ureteroscopes: a single center evaluation of the durability and function of the new endoscopes smaller than 9Fr. *J Urol* **164(4):** 1164–8

Anderson KR, Keetch DW *et al* (1994) Optimal therapy for the distal ureteral stone: extracorporeal shock wave lithotripsy versus ureteroscopy. *J Urol* **152(1):** 62–5

Bagley DH, Huffman JL *et al* (1983) Combined rigid and flexible ureteropyeloscopy. *J Urol* **130(2):** 243–4

Bagley DH, Huffman JL *et al* (1987) Flexible ureteropyeloscopy: diagnosis and treatment in the upper urinary tract. *J Urol* **138(2):** 280–5

Basillote JB, Lee DI *et al* (2004) Ureteroscopes: flexible, rigid, and semirigid. *Urol Clin North Am* **31(1):** 21–32

Delvecchio FC, Auge BK *et al* (2003) Assessment of stricture formation with the ureteral access sheath. *Urology* **61(3):** 518–22

Desai MM, Desai MR *et al* (2004) Endopyeloplasty versus endopyelotomy versus laparoscopic pyeloplasty for primary ureteropelvic junction obstruction. *Urology* **64(1):** 16–21

Erturk E, Herrman E (1993). Extracorporeal shock wave lithotripsy for distal ureteral stones. *J Urol* **149(6):** 1425–6

Gerber GS, Kim J *et al* (2000) Retrograde ureteroscopic endopyelotomy for the treatment of primary and secondary ureteropelvic junction obstruction in children. *Tech Urol* **6(1):** 46–9

Grocela JA, Dretler SP (1997) Intracorporeal lithotripsy. Instrumentation and development. *Urol Clin North Am* **24(1):** 13–23

Hollenbeck BK, Schuster TG *et al* (2003) Identifying patients who are suitable for stentless ureteroscopy following treatment of urolithiasis. *J Urol* **170(1):** 103–6

Huffman JL (1989) Ureteroscopic injuries to the upper urinary tract. *Urol Clin North Am* **16(2):** 249–54

Huffman JL (1989) Ureteroscopy: a 10-year perspective. *Semin Urol* **7(1):** 54–7

Johnson DB, Pearle MS (2004). Complications of ureteroscopy. *Urol Clin North Am* **31(1):** 157–71

Johnston WK, III, Low RK *et al* (2004) The evolution and progress of ureteroscopy. *Urol Clin North Am* **31(1):** 5–13

Joshi HB, Stainthorpe A *et al* (2003) Indwelling ureteral stents: evaluation of symptoms, quality of life and utility. *J Urol* **169(3):** 1065–9

Kim HL, Gerber GS (2000) Use of ureteroscopy and holmium:yttrium-aluminum-garnet laser in the treatment of an infundibular stenosis. *Urology* **55(1):** 129–31

Kourambas J, Byrne RR *et al* (2001) Does a ureteral access sheath facilitate ureteroscopy? *J Urol* **165(3):** 789–93

Lingeman JE, Sonda LP *et al* (1986) Ureteral stone management: emerging concepts. *J Urol* **135(6):** 1172–4

Matsuoka K, Iida S *et al* (1999) Endoscopic lithotripsy with the holmium:YAG laser. *Lasers Surg Med* **25(5):** 389–95

Michel MS, Knoll T *et al* (2002) The URO Mentor: development and evaluation of a new computer-based interactive training system for virtual life-like simulation of diagnostic and therapeutic endourological procedures. *BJU Int* **89(3):** 174–7

Netto NR, Jr., Ikonomidis J *et al* (2001) Routine ureteral stenting after ureteroscopy for ureteral lithiasis: is it really necessary? *J Urol* **166(4):** 1252–4

Osther PJ, Geertsen U *et al* (1998) Ureteropelvic junction obstruction and ureteral strictures treated by simple high-pressure balloon dilation. *J Endourol* **12(5):** 429–31

Pearle MS, Nadler R *et al* (2001) Prospective randomized trial comparing shock wave lithotripsy and ureteroscopy for management of distal ureteral calculi. *J Urol* **166(4):** 1255–60

Peschel R, Janetschek G *et al* (1999) Extracorporeal shock wave lithotripsy versus ureteroscopy for distal ureteral calculi: a prospective randomized study. *J Urol* **162(6):** 1909–12

Segura JW, Preminger GM *et al* (1997) Ureteral Stones Clinical Guidelines Panel summary report on the management of ureteral calculi. The American Urological Association. *J Urol* **158(5):** 1915–21

Tawfiek ER, Liu JB *et al* (1998) Ureteroscopic treatment of ureteropelvic junction obstruction. *J Urol* **160(5):** 1643–6

Watterson JD, Beiko DT *et al* (2002) Randomized prospective blinded study validating acquistion of ureteroscopy skills using computer based virtual reality endourological simulator. *J Urol* **168(5):** 1928–32

Yip KH, Lee CW *et al* (1998) Holmium laser lithotripsy for ureteral calculi: an outpatient procedure. *J Endourol* **12(3):** 241–6

Zheng W, Denstedt JD (2000) Intracorporeal lithotripsy. Update on technology. *Urol Clin North Am* **27(2):** 301–13

CHAPTER 7

General complications of laparoscopic surgery

R Madeb, J Joseph

Laparoscopic surgery in any speciality can have complications of the surgery. If the surgeon and his team are trained to recognize complications, this is the first step. This will lower the rate of problems. This chapter highlights the main areas to focus on when thinking about this area

Introduction

With the advancement of laparoscopic familiarity, equipment and techniques, many classical open surgical procedures have since been superseded by laparoscopic procedures. In many cases, the laparoscopic approach has become the new gold standard and replaced many traditional open methods. It is of little doubt, that the advancement of laparoscopic equipment coupled with the patient-driven interest in minimally invasive surgery has allowed for a reduction in complication rates with laparoscopy. Nevertheless, there is a learning curve associated with laparoscopic surgery and the surgeon should be familiar with complications associated with this approach. The following chapter reviews the incidence, type and etiology of the complications reported globally over the past decade with specific emphasis on the general complications associated with laparoscopic surgery.

Incidence of general complications

Most of the data available concerning complications in laparoscopic surgery has been recorded from procedures performed mostly by gynecologists and general surgeons. The incidence of complications associated with laparoscopy is reported to be between 0.3 and 2.8% for major complications and between 1 and 4% for minor complications in gynecological procedures (Hulka *et al*, 1973; Chaberlain and Carron-Brown, 1978; Cushieri, 1980; Riedel *et al*, 1986; Peterson *et al*, 1990). The overall complication rate for cholecystectomy has been reported to be 5.2 % (Cushieri *et al*, 1991). In a survey conducted by Phillips *et al* it was reported that the complication rate was four times higher in operations where the performing physician had less than 100 procedures experience (Philips *et al*, 1975). Although a decade of urologic laparoscopy has elapsed, no single urological procedure even begins to be comparable in frequency to cholecystectomy or ovarian laparoscopic procedures. Consequently, the true incidence of complications in urologic laparoscopy has not been clearly identified. Currently, much of the information regarding the perisurgical complications in urology is derived from individual case series for specific procedures. Furthermore, as some laparoscopic procedures are still in the developmental or learning phase, the complication rate is not accurately reflective of the true incidence. Nevertheless, some series of laparoscopic complications have been reported for specific urologic procedures including pelvic lymph node dissection, nephrectomy, adrenalectomy and prostatectomy. Kozminski and associates reviewed 105 patients having undergone pelvic node dissection and showed an overall complication rate of 21% of which only three (2.6%) patients had to be converted to laparotomy (Kozminski *et al*, 1992). Kavoussi and associates reviewed 327 patients also having undergone pelvic node dissection and showed an intra-operative complication rate of 4.3% (Kavoussi *et al*, 1993). Complication rates for all types of nephrectomy range from 6–13%, with a conversion rate of 3% for simple nephrectomy and 16% for radical nephrectomy (Soulie *et al*, 2001). Multi-institutional series of laparoscopic adrenalectomy performed in Japan have reported a complication rate of 32% with a conversion rate of 3.8% (Matsuda *et al*, 2000). Guillonneau *et al*. have recently published the World's largest series of laparoscopic radical prostatectomy and reported an overall complication rate of 17.1% (Guillonneau *et al*, 2002). The overall mortality rate due to laparoscopy has been shown to be between 0.005 and 0.5 % (Mintz, 1977; Kane and Krejs, 1984).

General laparoscopic complications

The following article identifies the incidence, type and etiology of the complications seen in multiple articles in the surgical literature during the past decade. This chapter reviews the general complications seen during access, pneumoperitoneum and anesthesia. *Table 7.1* summarizes the general complications seen with laparoscopic procedures.

Injury entering abdomen

The first steps of any laparoscopic procedure are establishment of a pneumoperitoneum and insertion of trocars. Therefore, access-related complications are the first potential site for injury during laparoscopy. The severity of these injuries ranges from inconsequential punctures to fatal hemorrhages usually involving visceral or vascular structures. The insertion of the trocar and Veress needle is associated with the greatest risk of injury during laparoscopic surgical procedures.

Table 7.1: General complications of laparoscopic surgery

Trocar and Veress Needle Insertion
Vascular injuries

Visceral injuries

Pneumatic Complications
Emphysema

Pneumothorax

Pneumomediastinum

Tension pneumoperitoneum

Gas embolism

Cardiac rhythm disturbances

Surgical Technique
Mechanical injury

Thermal injury

Visceral injury

Anesthesia Considerations

Post-Laparoscopic Complications
Surgical scar hernia

Subcutaneous emphysema

Fluid collections

Wound infection and ecchymosis

Peritonitis and fistula formation

Deep vein thrombosis and thrombophlebitis

Post-operative bleeding

Shoulder pain

Prolonged ileus

Port-Site metastasis

Procedure-based surveys of laparoscopic access injuries have reported low injury rates varying from five per 10,000 to three per 1000 (Champault *et al*, 1996). Recently, an injury-based reporting system database has been developed for both American and European systems, which accrues data, that is injury based and not procedure based. This study revealed that access related injuries could be serious conferring a mortality of 13%, with bowel and retroperitoneal vascular injuries compromising 76% of all injuries in the process of establishing a primary port (Champault *et al*, 1996; Chandler *et al*, 2001). Injury to underlying structures is more common with the use of reusable trocars as opposed to the disposable models. This can be attributed to the fact that the disposable trocars require less force (nearly 50% less in one study) (Corson *et al*, 1989) for peritoneal entry and are designed with a safety shield that extends over the sharp tip after passing through the peritoneum (Nezhat *et al*, 1991). Various techniques have been used in order to decrease access related injuries. The most common technique used upon entering the abdomen has been lifting the peritoneum prior to Veress needle insertion. This maneuver increases the distance between the abdominal wall and the underlying structures thereby decreasing the chance for puncture.

The most common vascular injury caused by trocar or Veress needle insertion is damage to the inferior epigastric artery (McDonald *et al*, 1978; Wolf and Carroll, 1993; Champault *et al*, 1996). As it supplies the rectus abdominus muscle, the inferior epigastric artery is at risk during initial entrance to the abdomen and during procedures that need a lateral trocar placed. This is especially true in advanced cases where multiple ports are usually needed. If the inferior epigastric artery is punctured it is often easily tamponaded with the cannula. If necessary, a foley catheter can be passed through the port site and drawn back to tamponade the vessel. For more significant bleeding full thickness sutures can be placed. Since all subsequent trocars used are inserted under direct visualization, it is only the primary trocar and the Veress needle that typically cause such injuries. Furthermore, bleeding from the abdominal wall vessels due to the Veress or trocar insertion can be coagulated or sutured following the immediate insertion of the second trocar. More severe and life-threatening injuries can occur with direct puncture to the retroperitoneal vessels at the aortic bifurcation, vena cava, and iliac arteries. These usually occur as the Veress needle is blindly inserted in the non-insufflated peritoneal space. The first sign that a major vascular injury has occurred is blood aspirated through the insufflation needle. Although major vascular injuries are rare, if not recognized quickly, these injuries can result in a high degree of morbidity and even mortality (Corson *et al*, 1989; Nezhat *et al*, 1991; Wolf and Carroll, 1993; Champault *et al*, 1996; Chandler *et al*; 2001). Therefore, it is essential to recognize injury early and attempt appropriate vascular repair. In most cases the only way to control large abdominal vessel damage is to perform an immediate laparotomy. This is one of the main reasons why some laparoscopists perform every laparoscopic procedure in an operating room that is equipped and ready for open laparotomy and vascular repair. To minimize the risk when inserting the Veress needle a 45° angle of insertion is recommended. A steeper angle is associated with retroperitoneal injury and a shallower angle with pre-peritoneal placement and subcutaneous insufflation (McDonald *et al*, 1978; Corson *et al*, 1989; Nezhat *et al*, 1991; Wolf and Carroll, 1993; Champault *et al*, 1996; Chandler *et al*; 2001).

Visceral organ damage is most likely to occur during insertion of the Veress needle and trocar. As previously mentioned, it is safer to use the disposable trocar for both safety and ease of entry. If the Veress needle is inserted midline with the angle of entry at 45° and the direction toward the sacrum, chances of puncture are small. If the bowel or bladder is punctured with the Veress needle, it usually does not result in need for laparotomy due to the small caliber of the needle. It is possible to perform laparoscopic repair of the bowel or bladder if the injury is well visualized. If detected intraoperatively, the injury can usually be repaired with intracorporeal suturing. However, injury to the intestine or stomach is not detected as readily as an injury to a blood vessel which usually has a gush of blood brought forth. Therefore, many abdominal perforations can go undetected resulting in postoperative ileus and peritonitis. If bowel or bladder punctures are made with the trocar it may be necessary to repair the tear by open laparotomy using the trocar in place as a guide. To reduce the possibility of visceral organ damage, the surgeon should avoid areas where adhesions or scars may exist from previous surgeries. Overall, there is no fool proof method for access and the establishment of the primary port. By thoroughly and systematically learning safe and proper techniques the incidence of access related complications could be brought to a minimum.

A variety of techniques have been used in order to decrease access related injuries, including open access (Hasson technique) and the use of non-bladed trocars with endoscopic guided ports (Visiport).The safest system is the open access technique originally described by Hasson in 1974 (Hasson, 1974). Although the open technique can be used for any case, it is recommended to be used for patients with previous abdominal surgery, in cases where an establishment of a pneumoperitoneum has failed with a Veress needle, for thin patients and for pediatric laparoscopic procedures. As would be expected there are fewer reports of vascular and bowel injury with the open method. However, they have been described and laparoscopic surgeons should be familiar with both approaches (Penfield, 1985; Hanney *et al*, 1999).

The non-bladed trocars have helped to decrease vascular injuries when used with the endoscopic guidance (Melzer *et al*, 1995). Until this was done, the potential for injuries by blind passage after Veress insufflation would be higher. In addition, wound healing and associated complications are improved by using a non-bladed trocar.

When exiting the abdomen it is important to do so under visual guidance to monitor potential bleeding areas, and bowel or omental herniation. Port sites should all be closed at the fascial layer in children and if >10mm in adults, otherwise herniation may occur. However, non-bladed trocars need not be closed as their defect is only half the size of the trocar (Kolata *et al*, 1999; Venkatesh, 2002).

Pneumatic Complications

Failure to place the Veress needle in the peritoneal space can result in subcutaneous, pre-peritoneal, or omental emphysema, and accidental insufflation of the bowel. Insufflation injuries have an occurrence rate of 3.5% but are mostly of minor significance (Chaberlain and Carron-Brown, 1978; Esposito, 1973; Pring, 1983; Capelouto and Kavoussi, 1993). Subcutaneous emphysema results from carbon dioxide leakage around trocar insertion points and from failed Veress needle insertion resulting in placement above the abdominal fascia. This is usually of minor significance, however, it could result in a pneumothorax, pneumomediastinum or hypercarbia (Doctor and Hussain, 1973; Bard and Chen, 1990; Kalhan and Reancy, 1990; Kent, 1991). Accidental placement of the Veress needle into the pre-peritoneal fat results in pre-peritoneal subcutaneous emphysema. This is usually not discovered until visualization of pre-peritoneal fat is made. It is of minor consequence, although it does increase the distance the trocar has to pass through. Open trocar placement following air evacuation is the safest manner to deal with this complication (Capelouto and Kavoussi, 1993). If the Veress needle is accidentally placed in the bowel, insufflation will result in asymmetrical abdominal distention. Laparoscopic procedure should be aborted if trocars have not already been placed. If a prolonged high intra-abdominal pressure is maintained it is possible to cause tension pneumoperitoneum. The high pressure causes partial compression of the vena cava resulting in a decrease in venous return and in turn a decrease in the cardiac output. The high pressure can also cause rupture through weak points in the diaphragm or along the great vessels resulting in pneumothorax or pneumomediastinum (Doctor and Hussain, 1973; Kalhan *et al*, 1990). Movement of the diaphragm and ventilation pressures may also be affected by higher intra-abdominal pressure.

The incidence of gas embolism is relatively low. It has been reported to occur in one of 63845 cases, (Yacoub *et al*, 1982) or fifteen of 113253 cases, (Wadhwa *et al*, 1978) and in seven of 119430 in a study of women undergoing gynecological laparoscopy (Hynes and Marshall, 1992). Gas embolism can occur during insufflation, intraoperatively, or postoperatively. Monitoring of the patient and attention to initial Veress needle placement is paramount. Insufflation gas embolism is usually attributed to erroneous Veress needle placement (McKenzie, 1971; Kleppinger, 1974). Alternatively, it has been suggested that peritoneal adhesions from prior surgical procedures may rupture during insufflation causing gas embolism (Cottin *et al*, 1996). Intraoperative complications resulting in gas embolism include high intra-abdominal pressures leading to embolism via intravasation, manipulation of an Inferior Vena Cava (IVC) puncture (made during trocar insertion or by surgical instrument) and manipulation with high intra-abdominal pressures (O'Sullivan *et al*, 1998). Postoperative gas embolism is thought to be due to transperitoneal absorption of carbon dioxide traps in the venous system that is released later on (Root *et al*, 1978). Support for this theory has been shown by increase in peritoneal surface carbon dioxide measurements taken postoperatively (Seed *et al*, 1970; Mullet *et al*, 1993). Therefore, careful monitoring of a patient suspected of having a gas embolism include cardiac monitoring (arrhythmias are a common complication of gas embolism into the right atrium) end tidal CO_2, and frequent auscultation of heart sounds. Cardiac auscultation of a 'millwheel murmur' is classic for a gas embolism (Keith *et al*, 1974). It has been shown that the increase in end tidal CO_2 is an early indicator for early gas embolism detection (Shulman and Aronson, 1984; De Plater and Jones, 1989; Ostman *et al*, 1990; Greville *et al*, 1991). It is additionally important to monitor intraoperative CO_2 levels to watch for acid base disturbances due to hypercarbia. Since most laparoscopic surgery is performed under general anesthesia, it is easy to maintain normal CO_2 blood gas levels through serial blood gases, end tidal CO_2 monitoring and appropriate adjustment of mechanical ventilation. If CO_2 changes result in acid base disturbances they can also result in potentially life-threatening arrhythmias. In the event of a gas embolism during surgery, the procedure should be immediately halted, CO_2 insufflation stopped, NO_2 withheld and 100% O_2 given. The patient should be placed in the left lateral decubitus position (Durant's position) with the head down to allow any gas to move to the apex of the heart retarding gas flow into the pulmonary system (Alvaran *et al*, 1978). In severe cases cardiopulmonary resuscitation measures should be initiated including placement of a central line so that any gas can be drawn out. In addition, hyperbaric oxygen and cardiopulmonary bypass have been shown to be of use (McGrath *et al*, 1989; Grim *et al*, 1990; Diakun, 1991).

Cardiac rhythm disturbances can occur from hypercarbia, gas embolism, vagal responses to increased abdominal pressure, and peritoneal irritation (Brantley and Riley, 1988; Doyle and Mark, 1989; Myles, 1991). Gas embolism has produced various types of arrhythmias including bradycardia, asystole, and ventricular arrhythmias (Brantley and Riley, 1988; Cottin *et al*, 1996). Hypercarbia or metabolic acidosis can elicit life-threatening arrhythmias as well (Scott and Julian, 1972; Fishurne, 1978; Gordon and Lewis, 1988; Peterson *et al*, 1982). During insufflation, vagal stimulation from high abdominal pressures can produce a bradyarrhythmias including sinus bradycardia, nodal rhythms, and atrioventricular dissociation. These were shown in a study to represent up to 14% of arrhythmias occurring during laparoscopy (Myles, 1991). Further, it has been shown that the use of atropine before insufflation can reduce the occurrence of these vagal responses (Levinson, 1977).

Another common pneumoperitoneum-related complication is postoperative shoulder pain. The radiating shoulder pain is caused by irritation of the diaphragm by subphrenic residual CO_2 and is commonly seen in cases where a transperitoneal route is used. The best way to prevent this minor complication is making sure that all the CO_2 is extracted from the abdominal cavity. Maneuvers such as placing the patient in the extreme lateral and Trendelenburg position during desufflation are helpful in extracting the CO_2 from the subphrenic space.

Anesthesia considerations

The Center for Disease Control in the United States published a study attributing up to 33% of deaths associated with laparoscopic tubal ligation to anesthetic complications (Peterson *et al*, 1982). The padding and position of the patient should be carefully considered to prevent nerve palsies and postoperative orthopedic problems. Steep Trendelenburg positioning of the patient should caution the anesthesiologist to be sensitive with anesthetic agents that can relax the esophageal sphincter and increase risk of aspiration. The use of metaclopramide may improve gastric emptying and esophageal sphincter tone (Hasnain and Matjasko, 1991). Adjunct use of H_2 blockers will elevate the gastric pH (Hasnain and Matjasko, 1991).

Cardiac arrhythmias have been reported to occur in as many as 17% of laparoscopic procedures (Scott and Julian, 1972). The most common are premature supraventricular contractions, sinus tachycardia, and aberrant QRS conduction (Loffer and Pent, 1977). Those less common include premature ventricular beats, bigemeny, and fusion beats (Loffer and Pent, 1977). Hypercarbia can result in life-threatening cardiac arrythmias, and has been shown to increase circulating catecholamines (Price, 1960; Scott and Julian, 1972; Fishurne, 1978; Gordon and Lewis, 1988). It is also of note that inhalation anesthetics like halothane are also arrhythmogenic. During initial insufflation with CO_2, plasma levels of catecholamines were shown to rise further increasing the risk of cardiac dysrhythmias (Mikami *et al*, 1996).

Mask ventilation can result in hypoventilation, to which deaths have been attributed, due to inefficiency of ventilation (Fishurne, 1978). In addition mask ventilation can result in gastric distention increasing the risk of visceral organ damage by puncture with the Veress needle or trocar. The use of depolarizing neuromuscular blockers and positive pressure ventilation is ideal to reduce complication risks. Time dependent absorption of CO_2 gas from the peritoneal cavity can produce a relative hypercarbia and the necessary adjustments to minute ventilation should be made. Since there is compression of the chest cavity from pressure on the diaphragm, the FRC of the patient will be decreased. If a volume mode ventilatory cycle is used, one must be aware of higher airway pressures and the possible risk of barotrauma.

Conclusion

It is logical to assume that as more surgeons become familiar with the laparoscopic approach an ever-increasing number of surgical procedures will be performed by this approach. Moreover, more complex operations will be attempted and performed. Therefore, any surgeon who undertakes laparoscopic surgery should familiarize themselves with the potential complications associated with this minimally invasive technique.

Key points for *Chapter 7*

- A masked complication can be fatal, and thus a laparoscopic surgeon must always be overcautious perioperatively.
- Certified training decreases the rate of complications.
- Mentoring during operations reduces the rate of complications.
- Open access to any area lowers the risk of port site visceral injuries.
- Anesthetic complications are reduced by working closely with a well trained anethetist.
- Exiting the abdomen must be under vision and cutting port sites should be closed at the fascial layer.
- Blunt trocars are safer and are less likely to require suturing.
- Patient positioning and padding is crucial when surgeons are on the learning curve, as operation times are longer.

References

Alvaran SB, Toung JK *et al* (1978) Venous air embolism: comparative merits of external cardiac massage, intracardiac aspiration , and left lateral decubitus position. *Anesth Analg* **57**: 166–70

Bard PA, and Chen L (1990) Subcutaneous emphysema associated with laparoscopy. *Anesth Analg* **71**: 101–2

Brantley JC and Riley PM (1988) Cardiovascular collapse during laparoscopy: a report of two cases. *Am J Obstet Gynecol* **159**: 735–7

Capelouto CC, and Kavoussi LR (1993) Complications of Laparoscopic Surgery. *Urology* **42(1)**: 2–12

Chaberlain GVP and Carron-Brown J (1978) *Gynaecological Laparoscopy*, Royal College of Obstetricians and Gynaecologists, London.

Champault G, Cazacu F *et al* (1996) Serious trocar accidents in laparoscopic surgery: a French survey of 103852 operations. *Surg Laparosc Endosc* **6(5)**: 367–70

Chandler JG, Corson SL *et al* (2001) Three spectra of laparoscopic entry access injuries. *J Am Coll Surg* **192(4)**: 478–91

Corson SL, Batzer FR *et al* (1989) Measurement of force necessary for laparoscopic trocar entry. *J Reprod Men* **34**: 282–4

Cottin V, Delafosse B *et al* (1996) Gas embolism during laparoscopy. *Surg Endosc* **10**: 166–9

Cushieri A, Dubois F *et al* (1991) The European experience with laparoscopic cholecystectomy. *Am J Surg* **161**: 385–7

Cushieri A (1980) Laparoscopy in general surgery and gastroenterology. *Br J Hosp Med* **24**: 255–8

De Plater RM, Jones IS (1989) Non fatal carbon dioxide embolism during laparoscopy. *Anaesth Intensive Care* **17**: 359–61

Diakun TA (1991) Carbon dioxide embolism: successeful rescusitation with cardiopulmonary bypass. *Anesthesiology* **74**: 1151–3

Doctor NH, Hussain Z (1973) Bilateral pneumothorax associated with laparoscopy: a case report of a rare hazard and review of the literature. *Anesthesia* **28**: 75–81

Doyle DJ, Mark PW (1989) Laparoscopy and vagal arrest (Letter). *Anesthesia* **44**: 448

Esposito JM (1973) Hematoma of the sigmoid colon as a complication of laparoscopy. *Am J Obstet Gynecol* **117**: 581–2

Fishurne JI (1978) Anesthesia for laparoscopy: considerations , complications, and techniques. *J Reprod Med* **21**: 37–40

Gordon AG, Lewis BV (1982) In: *Gynecological Endoscopy*, JB Lippincott, Philadelphia

Greville AC, Clements EA *et al* (1991). Pulmonary air embolism during laparoscopic laser cholecystectomy. *Anaesthesia* **46**: 113–4

Grim PS, Gottlieb LJ *et al* (1990) Hyperbaric oxygen therapy. *J Am Med Assoc* **263**: 2216–20

Guillonneau B, Rozet F *et al* (2002) Perioperative complications of laparoscopic radical prostatectomy: the Montsouris 3-year experience. *J Urol* **167(1):** 51–6

Hanney RM, Carmalt HL *et al* (1999) Vascular injuries during laparoscopy associated with the Hasson technique. *J Am Coll Surg* **188(3):** 337–8.

Hasnain JU, Matjasko MJ (1991) Practical anesthesia for laparoscopic surgeries. In Zucker KA (ed) *Surgical Laparoscopy.* Quality Medical Publishing, St. Louis 77–86

Hasson HM (1974) open lap: a report of 150 cases. *J Reprod Med* **12:** 234–8

Hulka JF, Soderstrom RM *et al* (1973) Complications committee of the American Associations of Gynecologic Laparoscopists, First annual report. *J Reprod Med* **10:** 301–6

Hynes SR, Marshall RL (1992) Venous gas embolism during gynecological laparoscopy. *Can J Anesth* **39:** 748–9

Kalhan SB, Reaney JA (1990) Pneumomediastinum and subcutaneous emphysema during laparoscopy. *Cleve Clin J Med* **57:** 639–42

Kane MG, Krejs GJ (1984) Complications of diagnostic laparoscopy in Dallas: a 7-year prospective study. *Gastointest Endosc* **30:** 237–40

Kavoussi LR, Sosa E, Chandhoke P *et al* (1993) Complications of laparoscopic pelvic lymph node dissection. *J Urol* **149:** 322–5

Keith L, Silver A *et al* (1974) Anesthesia for laparoscopy. *J Reprod Med* **12:** 227–33

Kent RB (1991) Subcutaneous emphysema and hypercarbia following laparoscopic cholecytectomy. *Arch Surg* **126:** 1154–6

Kleppinger RK (1974) One thousand laparoscopies of a community hospital. *J Reprod Med* **13:** 13–20

Kolata RJ, Ransick M *et al* (1999) Comparison of wounds created by non-bladed trocars and pyramidal tip trocars in the pig. *J Laparoendosc Adv Surg Tech A* **9:** 455–61

Kozminski M, Gomella L *et al* (1992) Laparoscopic urologic surgery: outcome assessment (Abstract 127) *J Urol* **147:** 245A

Levinson CJ (1977) Complications. In: Phillips JM (ed): *Laparoscopy.* Williams & Wilkins, Baltimore 220–30

Loffer FD, Pent D (1977) Statistics. In Phillips JM (Ed): *Laparoscopy.* Williams & Wilkins, Baltimore 243–6

Matsuda T, Kawakita M *et al* (2000) Future of urologic laparoscopy. *World J Surg* **24(10):** 1172–5

McDonald PT, Rich NM *et al* (1978) Vascular trauma secondary to diagnostic and therapeutic procedures: laparoscopy. *Am J Surg* **135:** 651–5

McGrath RB, Zimmerman JE *et al* (1989) Carbon dioxide embolism treated with hyperbaric oxygen. *Can J Anaesth* **36:** 586–9

McKenzie R (1971) Laparoscopy. *NZ Med J* **74:** 87–91

Melzer A, Riek S *et al* (1995) Endoscopically controlled trocar and cannula insertion. *Endosc Surg Allied Technol* **3:** 63–8

Mikami O, Kawakita S *et al* (1996) Catecholamine release caused by carbon dioxide insufflation during laparoscopic surgery. *J Urol* **155:** 1368–71

Mintz M (1977) Risks and prophylaxis in laparoscopy: a survey of 100,000 cases. *J Reprod Med* **18:** 269–72

Mullet CE, Viale JP *et al* (1993) Pulmonary CO2 elimination during surgical procedures using intra or extraperitoneal CO_2 insufflation. *Anesth Analg* **76:** 622–6

Myles PS (1991) Bradyarrythmias and laparoscopy: a prospective study of heart rate changes with laparoscopy. *Aust NZ J Obstet Gynaecol* **31:** 171–3

Nezhat FR, Silfen SL *et al* (1991) Comparison of direct insertion of disposable and standard reusable laparoscopic trocars and previous pneumoperitoneum with Veress needle. *Obstet Gynecol* **78:** 148–50

O'Sullivan DC, Micali S *et al* (1998) Factors involved in gas embolism after laparoscopic injury to inferior vena cava. *J Endourol* **12(2):** 149–54

Ostman PL, Pantle Fisher FH *et al* (1990) Circulatory Collapse during laparoscopy. *J Clin Anesth* **2:** 129–32

Penfield AJ (1985) How to prevent complications of open laparoscopy. *J Reprod Med* **30(9):** 660–3.

Peterson HB, DeStefano F *et al* (1982) Deaths attributable to tubal sterilization in the United States, 1977–1981. *Am J Obstet Gynecol* **146:** 131–6

Peterson HB, Hulka JF *et al* (1990) American Association of Gynecological Laparoscopists' 1988 membership survey on operative laparoscopy. *J Reprod Med* **35:** 587–9

Phillips J, Keith D *et al* (1975) Survey of Gynecological laparoscopy for 1974. *J Reprod Med* **15:** 45–50

Price HL (1960) Efects of carbon dioxide on the cardiovascular system. *Anesthesiology* **21:** 652

Pring DW (1983) Inferior epigastric hemmorrhage: an avoidable complication of laparoscopic clip sterilization. *Br J Obstet Gynaecol* **90:** 480–2

Riedel HH, Lehmann-Willenbrock E *et al* (1986) German pelviscopic statistics for the years 1978–1982. *Endoscopy* **18:** 219–22

Root B, Levy MN *et al* (1978) Gas embolism death after laparoscopy delayed by 'trapping' in portal circulation. *Anesth Analg* **57:** 232–7

Scott DB, Julian DG (1972) Observations on cardiac arrythmias during laparoscopy. *Br Med J* **1:** 411–3

Seed RF, Shakespeare TF *et al* (1970) Carbon dioxide homeostasis during anesthesia for laparoscopy. *Anaesthesia* **25:** 223–31

Shulman D, Aronson HB (1984) Capnography in the early diagnosis of carbon dioxide embolism during laparoscopy *Can Anaesth Soc J* **31:** 455–9

Soulie M, Seguin P *et al* (2001) Urological complications of laparoscopic surgery: experience with 350 procedures at a single center. *J Urol* **165(6 Pt 1):** 1960–3

Wadhwa RK, McKenzie R *et al* (1978) Gas embolism during laparoscopy. *Anesthesiology* **48:** 74–6

Wolf SJ, Carroll P (1993) Laparoscopic access to and exit from the abdomen. *Atlas Urol Clin North Am* **1(2):** 1–15

Yacoub OF, Cardona I *et al* (1982) Carbon dioxide embolism during laparoscopy. *Anesthesiology* **57:** 533–5

CHAPTER 8

Training surgeons in laparoscopic surgery

SKH Yip, CWS Cheng

Laparoscopic techniques are developing rapidly and their application is widespread. Structured laparoscopic training is recommended and desirable, for both trainee and practicing surgeons. Training models include inanimate skill training, including pelvic trainer or virtual reality. Specific skills (tasks) are practiced in preparation for live surgery. Cadaveric dissection and live animal surgery training, where available, allow appreciation of surgical anatomy and practice of tissue handling. The latter, in particular, demands the integration of laparoscopic skills, judgement and operating room management simulating live surgery. It is invaluable in skill acquisition and development of procedures.

The above training modalities, combined with appropriate courses and hands-on experience under supervision, form the framework of training. Practical experience and critical review will continue to enhance the skill. National bodies should take the lead to recommend appropriate training programs to enhance improved patient outcome

Introduction

Traditional surgical skills training are largely based on a mentor-apprenticeship system. The axiom 'see one, do one, teach one' was taken for granted. Training activities revolved around the operating room (OR) and real 'cases', and different types of surgery require different skill sets (*Table 8.1*). However, such training is time consuming and labor intensive. The increased operating time also has significant cost implications, reported as a cost of US$ 47970 per graduating surgical resident (Bridges and Diamond, 1999). In addition to cost consideration, there are ethical as well as medico-legal implications. Importantly, such apprenticeship systems rely largely on subjective assessment, where a 'graduated' surgeon will make an assessment and re-certification. This poses a tremendous challenge for patient care when trying to train and re-validate surgeons.

The rapid development of new surgical skills and technology particularly for practicing urologists, means ongoing training methods which limit the risk to patients are essential. In a survey conducted by Best *et al*, residents who were exposed to laparoscopy training would typically offer minimally invasive surgery for suitable candidates because of the obvious benefits of reduced pain and hospital stay. Alternatively, those who graduated before the laparoscopy era were much less likely to offer such treatment despite the obvious advantages of MIS (Best *et al*, 2002).

Is there a need for laparoscopy training?

Laparoscopic surgery involves very different visual conception and hand-eye co-ordination compared to conventional open surgery. This is related to the use of different instruments, relative lack of tactile sensation, the limited range of movement and the fulcrum effect which makes movements counter intuitive.

In 1991 Clayman *et al* performed the first laparoscopic nephrectomy (Clayman *et al*, 1991). But it had taken a long while for laparoscopic urology to become commonplace. One possibility could be that there is no simple urological operation compared to laparoscopic cholecystectomy or fallopian tube ligation. The entry level is 'nephrectomy' for laparoscopic urology, which more often than not involves abnormal anatomy from cancers. Despite the above, ablative procedures including laparoscopic nephrectomy for both benign and malignant disease, and subsequently live donor nephrectomy were increasingly practiced and accepted as gold standard. Reconstructive procedures, such as laparoscopic pyeloplasty, laparoscopic partial nephrectomy and laparoscopic radical prostatectomy soon followed this trend of minimally invasive surgery. It is interesting to note even Clayman's group at one time felt, but did not publish the fact that laparoscopic prostatectomy was just too difficult. A few years later, the French revolutionized this field with groundbreaking results of laparoscopic radical prostatectomy (Mounsouris). To add to this, robotic assisted laparoscopic prostatectomy allowed laparoscopically naïve surgeons to perform this advanced surgery.

With all these rapid developments, the push to jump on the bandwagon, sometimes without adequate preparation and training, could have fuelled the higher incidence of complications. In a study conducted by Rosser *et al* addressing skill acquisition and assessment for laparoscopic surgery, it is astonishing to find that for ninety-six board-certified surgeons, 57% required >5 minutes to complete a stitch while 82% took either >5 minutes or could not complete a knot in <10minutes (Rosser *et al*, 1997). Interestingly, after the relevant instructions were given regarding suturing technique, the time required declined significantly and continued to improve with practice.

Obviously, there is a paradigm shift in surgical education. It is desirable to have standardization of surgical skills acquisition. Performance needs to be assessed in a uniform setting and programs need to be developed to ensure maintenance of surgical skills as well as acquisition of new surgical skills.

Inanimate skills training

The McGill Inanimate System for Training and Evaluation of Laparoscopic Skills (MISTELS) and Yale laparoscopic skills and suturing program were assessed in 1998 (Derossis *et al*, 1998; Rosser *et al*, 1998). Such systems can be installed with relative ease. They allow unlimited practice and little supervision is required after the initial instructions. It is relatively cheap but no live tissue or anatomy is involved.

Table 8.1: Skill sets and features of different surgical modalities

Mode	Features	Typical procedures	Remarks
Traditional open surgery	3-dimensional and tactile sensation	Radical nephrectomy retropubic prostatectomy	Decreasing availability of good 'teaching' cases, increasing inclincation to offer minimally invasive surgery
Endoscopic surgery	Monocular view and reduced tactile sensation	TURP, URS, PCNL	Essential and integral part of of modern day urology practice, urologists pioneered endo-surgery
Laparoscopic surgery (ablative)	2-dimentional and reduced tactile sensation	Radical nephrectomy donor nephrectomy	'Entry' level much more demanding, adoption of laparoscopy technique lags behind general surgery
Laparoscopic surgery (reconstructive)	2-dimentional and reduced tactile sensation	Radical prostatectomy partial nephrectomy	Highly demanding, often involves a hybrid of technology and technique\
Lap prostatectomy set new milestone in lap urology
Robotic-assisted laparoscopy	3-dimentional (computer generated) no tactile sensation	Robot assisted lap prostatectomy robot-assisted pyeloplasty	Intuitive, overcomes difficulty in reconstructive procedures, highly costly, not readily accessible

TURP – transurethral resection of prostate; URS – ureteroscopy; PCNL – percutaneous nephrolithotomy

The effectiveness of transfer of technique

Fried *et al* evaluated twelve residents randomized to MISTEL training and no training control (Fried *et al*, 1999). A series of seven analogue skills were then tested in an in-vivo porcine model. It was noted that there was significant improvement over control in cutting, clipping, mesh placement as well as suturing. An even more interesting study was reported by Scott (2001). Nine residents were trained in Yale skill program, thirty minutes per day for ten days (twenty-eight times for each task). Their performance in subsequent clinical laparoscopic surgery and that of control residents were assessed by three independent expert surgeons where scores were assigned regarding different aspects. It was found that the trained group achieved greater median improvement in operating room performance and better overall performance. (Scott *et al*, 2001) From the above two studies, it may be concluded that skills acquired on a laparoscopic simulator are transferable to in-vivo (animal) surgery and more importantly, to actual operating room setting.

However, Scott also noted that the performance (time in seconds for task) reached a plateau at thirty to thirty-five repetitions. It may be extrapolated that such inanimate training is good for beginners. Beyond a certain limit, the skills may not progress despite repetitive training.

Various bench models are available commercially, some of which simulate pelvic pathology and allow for practice including 'urethro-vesical anastomosis' after radical prostatectomy. These may be good models to be installed in ORs, staff rooms or offices to facilitate in-house staff training at their convenience. Residents can be requested to log their practice sessions or the performance being videotaped to ensure completion of tasks within certain time frames.

Virtual reality

Drawing on the successful paradigm of flight simulation, Satava first proposed training surgical skills in virtual reality in 1993 (Satava, 1993). Surgical tasks that are inefficient, impractical, slow, costly or even dangerous if taught in the operating room may be best learned during an analog experience before coming to the operating room.

The computer generated environment mimics reality by combining physical models and realistic interfaces. The simulation can be skill, task or procedure based. However, for more complex procedures, the discrepancy between life and virtual reality may become more pronounced. Currently, available systems include minimally invasive surgery training virtual reality (MIST-VR) by Mentice, Lap Sim by Surgical Science and Lap-mentor by Symbionus where specific procedure and case scenario are available.

The virtual reality-training platform allows unlimited practice. Errors and progress can be assessed while the level of difficulty can be adjusted. However, drawbacks include the absence of tactile sensation and the use of non-real instruments.

Questions remain as to how closely the actual operation is being simulated. In the landmark paper by Seymour where sixteen surgical residents were randomized to MIST-VR training and no training, their performance of laparoscopic cholecystectomy were subject to two experts blinded to randomization. The trained group performed the gall bladder dissection 29% faster while the untrained group had significantly higher incidence of transient failure to progress (nine times), injury of gall bladder (five times) and burning non-target tissue (five times). Mean errors were six times less likely in the VR trained group. This validation of transfer of training skills from VR to OR sets the stage for more sophisticated use of VR in assessment, training, error reduction and re-certification of surgeons (Seymour *et al*, 2002).

A recent study by Grantcharov *et al* again examined the impact of VR surgical simulation on improvement of psychomotor skills relevant to the performance of laparoscopic cholecystectomy. Twenty residents with little laparoscopic experience were randomized to ten repetitions of six tasks on MIST-VR or no training. It was noted that trained residents had a significantly shorter procedure time, less errors and more economy of movements. It was concluded that VR surgical simulation can be a valid tool for training of laparoscopic psychomotor skills (Grantcharov *et al*, 2004). Whether VR is more efficient than inanimate simulation is debatable. Clinical scenarios can be built in a VR environment to enhance the skill/ task training to include judgement training. On the other hand, a pelvic trainer setting may incorporate wet tissue handling and has the advantages of tactile feedback on tissue.

The adoption of flight simulation by the aviation industry and government is fast and considered cost-worthy for obvious reasons. However, a clinical skills training simulator faces different challenges. The capital investment of individual service units training a handful of surgical residents per year may seem undesirable. It may be worth academic or training bodies sharing the cost of such devices for a bigger common pool and a constant flow of surgical trainees. It must be remembered that the skills improvement may plateau off as in inanimate laparoscopy training.

An interesting study by Mackay *et al* studied forty-one novice subjects for training in time blocks of twenty minutes or four time blocks each of five minutes. The latter group scored better for time, error and economy of movement (Mackay *et al*, 2002). The dictum of 'practice makes perfect' may therefore be amended to 'practice, rest and more practice make perfection'.

Cadaver dissection training

In this setting, real anatomy is appreciated but tissue responses are absent. Availability is limited and can be costly. Due to the underlying sensitivity, such programs may not be widely available. Even then, training centres may not advertise extensively for obvious reasons. However, it obviously provides one of the best models for understanding the anatomy before contemplating laparoscopic complex surgery. It is far superior to animal based models. For example in the porcine model the bladder is largely intra-abdominal while the urethra hangs freely in a wide pelvis, which is not the case when performing the urethra-vesical anastomosis in human radical prostatectomy.

Wet laboratory training

The live animal training set up provides a platform for integration of skills training, on site judgement and co-ordination of facility and personnel. While details of anatomy differ from humans, the upper urinary tract of the porcine model does bear significant similarity to a human setting.

The respect of a live subject, the desirability of avoiding error and a favorable outcome especially in non-acute animal reversal experiments, dictate a cautious effort by the trainees to take the training seriously. The operating environment is also similar to the OR, where instruments can fail and efforts need to be coordinated. This type of integrated training is not available in most of the other systems mentioned above.

For complex surgery or new procedures, the training of a team of surgeons, assistants and even nurses is invaluable as exemplified in our introduction of the live donor nephrectomy program (Chiong *et al*, 2004). However, it is a costly and labor-intensive exercise. There are also animal rights concerns and cultural sensitivity involved. It is important that training requirements and study protocol follow individual institute as well as the country's requirements. Appropriate approval from the institute's animal care committee is mandatory.

Courses and mentorship

The availability of video and computer technology allows unique opportunity for performances to be reviewed, studied, criticized and improved upon. Real life operation provides the best platform in learning. Yet, review of performance avoids repeating errors subsequently. A critique-review system may be incorporated in clinical training programs. Also, anatomy has been visualized like never before and images of entire operative procedures can be reproduced and used as teaching material on a self-learning basis. Many experts are generous enough to distribute their unique ways of performing certain procedures in a non-commercial, educational setting including VCD, DVD or over the internet.

Basic and advanced laparoscopy training courses are becoming widely available. Certain training programs and accreditation require mandatory attendance and certification. In fact, a very reasonable algorithm involving attendance of basic and advanced courses was recently proposed (*Figure 8.1*). Between which, there should be sufficient independent practice of skills as well as practical experience of assisting a mentor at laparoscopic procedure (McNeil and Tolley, 2002).

The spread of robotic assisted prostatectomy adds a new perspective to our understanding of training which obviously is not limited to residents in training. Menon *et al* and Ahlering *et al*, respectively demonstrated that laparoscopic 'naive' but well versed 'open' surgeons can readily acquire new technology

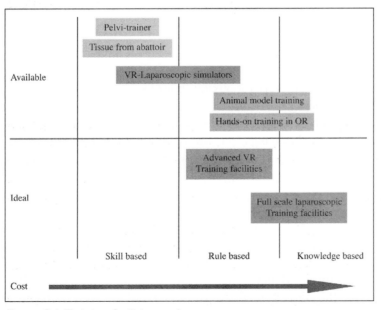

Figure 8.1: Training facilities and cost

Table 8.2: Training for man-machine system

Behaviour level	Activities	Facilities
SBB Skills Based Behaviour	Handling of surgical instruments Basic handling of tissue	Pelvi-trainer, Simple VR simulators, Tissue from abbattoirs
RBB Rule Based Behaviour	Learning protocols. Realistic tissue handling	Books, Courses, Lectures
KBB Knowledge Based Behaviour	Handling of unexpected events and of unknown symptoms. Decision making of complex tasks	Training on animal models, Hands on training in the operation theatre

and incorporate the new skills (Menon *et al*, 2002; Ahlering *et al*, 2003). Indeed, the man-machine interface is an exciting phenomenon and novel proposition, however the training pathway would be similar to other machine operations (*Table 8.2*).

It is interesting to note from Ahlering's report that the number of cases required to acquire the robotic skill is not tremendous. This is probably partly related to the clear demonstration of entire procedures and establishment of standard approach and partly in relation to the intuitive nature of the robot system. Proctorship is also recognized in robotic assisted prostatectomy. Our experience suggests that proctoring for three to five cases seems adequate for introduction of a robotic program, assuming the other factors including a dedicated team, availability of experienced laparoscopic assistants and a constant flow of suitable patients have been fulfilled (Sim and Yip, 2004).

Why do we want to train?

The reasons to train despite the cost, time and resource investment may not be easy to condense into one simple sentence. There is just a natural inclination to teach in the medical fraternity.

There are numerous models of world-renowned laparoscopy as well as robotic surgery training centers. Some are even commercially profitable. Yet, the development of new technologies and techniques is just too rapid. It is important that national bodies and academic units work closely to avoid duplication or undue competition to 'offer' training.

Training would be more beneficial if there is a concerted and coordinated effort targeted for incoming trainees as well as practicing urologists in the community. There should also be an unbiased collaboration with commercial vendors so that new devices and technologies have the appropriate platform.

Established and advanced institutes and countries should offer their expertise to less advanced countries so that the standard of care progression is global.

Conclusion

There is an urgent need to standardize surgical training including laparoscopic urology. While the problem has been defined, the tools and the programs are already available; there remains a need for validation of the curriculum. Currently, work in the field is in progress and validated programs may be used for further certification.

The authors want to acknowledge the invaluable input to the preparation of this manuscript by Dr Francis Lee, University of Hong Kong Medical Center and Dr David Albala of Duke University Medical Center.

Key points for *Chapter 8*

- The laparoscopic approach is increasingly accepted in a wide range of urology practice. In some areas, it has become the preferred modality, if not the standard of care.

- Ablative urology procedure, eg. laparoscopic nephrectomy, is technically demanding; and reconstructive urology, eg. laparoscopic prostatectomy is even more challenging.

- There is rapid development of laparoscopy technique, as well as evolution of technology.

- Laparoscopic surgery requires a different set of skills, fairly different from conventional open surgery, both residents and practising urologist need to go through proper and structured training to acquire the necessary skills.

- Inanimate training, eg. pelvic trainer, is a good platform from which to acquire the initial skills in laparoscopic surgery, and in certain instances, certain specific tasks including 'vesico-urethral' anastomosis.

- Virtual reality, in addition to 'skill' training, can be utilized to train on 'entire' procedures with varying degrees of difficulty. Scoring system are available for objective assessment, scenarios can be rehearsed to prepare for anticipated life situation.

- Cadaveric dissection training, where available, allows for appreciation of surgical anatomy.

- Live animal surgery requires the integration of surgical skills including tissue handling, 'clinical' judgement and OR management. It is invaluable for acquisition of skills and development of the surgical team.

- Courses and supervised hands-on training are integral parts of the training. Videos and computerized technology allow for mentoring and critical review of performance.

- National bodies should take the lead in recommending structured training programs and requirements for re-certification.

References

Ahlering TE, Skarecky D *et al* (2003) Successful transfer of open surgical skills to a laparoscopic environment using a robotic interface: initial experience with laparoscopic radical prostatectomy. *J Urol* **170(5):** 1738–41.

Best S, Erecole B *et al* (2004) Minimally invasive therapy for renal cell carcinoma: is there a community standard? *Urology* **64(1):** 22–5

Bridges M, Diamond DL (1999) The financial impact of teaching surgical residents in the operation room. *Am J Surg* **177(1):** 28–32

Chiong E, Yip SK *et al* (2004) Hand-assisted laparoscopic living donor nephrectomy. *Ann Acad Med Singapore* **33(3):** 294–7

Clayman RV, Kavoussi LR *et al* (1991) Laparoscopic nephrectomy: initial case report. *J Urol* **146(2):** 278–82.

Derossis AM, Fried GM *et al* (1998) Development of a model for training and evaluation of laparoscopic skills. *Am J Surg* **175(6):** 482–7

Fried GM, Derossis AM *et al* (1999) Comparison of laparoscopic performance in vivo with performance measured in a laparoscopic simulator. *Surg Endosc* **13(11):** 1077–81

Grantcharov TP, Kristiansen VB *et al* (2004) Randomized clinical trial of virtual reality simulation for laparoscopic skills training. *BJS* **91:** 146–50

Mackay S, Morgan P *et al* (2002) Practice distribution in procedural skills training: a randomized controlled trial. *Surg Endosc* **16(6):** 957–61

McNeil SA, Tolley DA (2002) Laparoscopy in urology: indication and training. *BJU Int* **89(3):** 169–73

Menon M, Shrivastava A *et al* (2002) Laparoscopic and robot assisted radical prostatectomy: establishment of a structured program and preliminary analysis of outcomes. *J Urol* **168(3):** 945–9.

Rosser JC, Rosser LE *et al* (1998) Objective evaluation of a laparoscopic surgical skill program for residents and senior surgeons. *Arch Surg* **133(6):** 657–61

Rosser JC, Rosser LE *et al* (1997) Skill acquisition and assessment for laparoscopic surgery. *Arch Surg* **132(2):** 200–04

Satava RM (1993). Virtual reality surgical simulator. The first steps. *Surg Endosc* **7(3):** 203–5

Scott DJ, Young WN *et al* (2001) Laparoscopic skills training. *Am J Surg* **182(2):** 137–42

Seymour NE, Gallagher AG *et al* (2002) Virtual reality training improves operating room performance results of a randomized, double-blined study. *Ann Surg* **236(4):** 458–63

Sim HG, Yip SK (2004) Early experience with robot-assisted laparoscopic radical prostatectomy. *Asian J Surg* **27(4):** 321–5

CHAPTER 9

Minimally invasive surgery: the economic impact

EC Ray, LO Schoeniger

Minimally invasive surgery has challenged traditional surgical paradigms and has become the preferred approach to a number of diseases. Before universal acceptance, any new procedure or technology should be critically analyzed with respect to its *safety, clinical utility, effectiveness* and *cost*. Laparoscopic cholecystectomy met all of these tests while reducing the cost and risk associated with the treatment of gallbladder disease. Calculating the 'cost' of any procedure, in the broadest sense, should include not only operating room expenses and the price of hospitalization, but also the cost to the individual and society. Reduced morbidity and shorter recovery periods translate into improved productivity, a component of 'cost' that is difficult to quantify. Minimally invasive procedures are typically less painful and more cosmetically satisfying. In an era where the cost of healthcare is spiraling ever higher, third party payers and government agencies have imposed measures to control healthcare expenditures, placing constraints on providers and consumers around the world. As a result of the new cost-containment environment, cost is increasingly seen as a measurable outcome of medical treatments. Society must weigh available technology and the preferences of the patient against limited healthcare resources.

Introduction

Minimally invasive surgery, particularly laparoscopic surgery, has challenged the paradigms of traditional surgical care, leading medicine as a whole to analyze what constitutes the 'standard of care.' Whenever a new technology emerges on the medical front, whether it is a medication, procedure or instrument, several issues should be addressed in order to effectively assess its utility. One should question the clinical need, the safety, the effectiveness and the cost. The availability of a new tool does not automatically justify its use. While the need, safety and efficacy of new technology validate its utility in a theoretical sense, the cost (to the individual, to the healthcare provider and to society) must be affordable.

Soon after fiber optics became available to the surgical practitioner in the 1970's, the potential benefits and applications of the technology became apparent (Bloom *et al*, 1973). In this regard, clinical need refers to the applicability of the new technology to the general population. Early in the development of new tools, procedures or medications, the subset of patients that will most benefit from the technology should be identified. Subsequently, trials are undertaken to test the new technology against a gold standard (a drug or procedure that is deemed to be the most effective). Before being introduced to the medical world, the new technology must be tested for safety. Next, the efficacy of the technology is evaluated. After the appropriate testing and approval, the final hurdle to routine application of a medical contrivance is affordability.

With the explosion of medical technology and an aging, underinsured population, the world has entered an era of healthcare cost-containment. This has been accomplished in both socialized (eg United Kingdom) and privatized medical cultures by limiting access to expensive procedures and treatments. The gatekeepers, whether government entities or private insurers, evaluate available treatments and set reimbursements for each to avoid excessive costs.

The field of Surgery is now facing these realities and actively participating in the evaluation of technologies by comparing the old to the new. When it comes to cost, the issue transcends hospital bills and professional fees. This section looks at what constitutes the cost of minimally invasive surgery and what economic impact the emerging technology may have on medicine as a whole.

The introduction of laparoscopic cholecystectomy by Phillipe Mouret in 1987 (Mouret, 1990) exemplifies a point in medical history where technology fulfilled a great role in not only reducing pain and suffering but in revolutionizing the way the public expected healthcare to be delivered. Patients left the hospital sooner and with fewer complications. Elective operations were performed in a shorter time period. A new gold standard emerged, as shown by the rapid diffusion of this procedure soon after its introduction (*Figure 9.1*) This has not been the case for all laparoscopic procedures, and in some cases the technology still seems to be searching for a justification of its application (Hopkins, 2000; Taner *et al*, 2001).

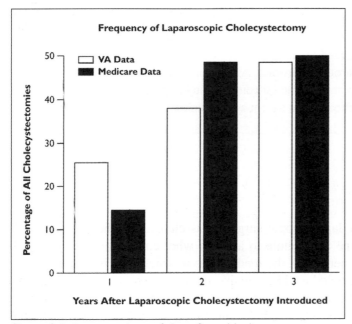

Figure 9.1: A comparison of data from Medicare and the Veterans Administration: the percentage of all cholecystectomies that were performed using the laparoscopic technique during the first three years after the procedure was introduced (Nenner et al, 1994; Ferreira et al, 1999).

When measuring the true cost of a medical device, there are numerous components that must be considered, many of which are very difficult to quantify. First, there is the cost of the operation itself. Second, there is the cost of the hospital stay, which usually correlates with the length of stay. Third, there is the overall cost, which includes expenditures for convalescence, follow-up and any potential complications or morbidity that leads to further healthcare utilization.

In the operating room (OR), there are many ways that a new procedure will impact cost. For one, the time for the operation will impact upon the cost of anesthesia and the operating room 'overhead' costs such as lighting, equipment maintenance and OR staff. One can think of time spent in the OR as a taxi driver's meter that is always running – the longer the operative time, the greater the price tag of the operation. The time it takes for surgeons and surgeons-in-training to learn new minimally invasive techniques translates into longer operating times. Even in experienced hands, laparoscopic procedures often take longer than open procedures, though this is not universally true. In addition, surgical instruments (purchase, cleaning and repairs) and other hardware needed to keep the OR running add to the overall cost. Special monitors, cameras, electrocautery, lighting and video controls are necessary to perform laparoscopic procedures. Disposable equipment adds additional cost when compared to reusable instruments. Some cost analyses have concluded that by eliminating disposable tools and reducing operative times, the financial burden of laparoscopic surgery can be reduced to the level of conventional open operations (Link *et al*, 2004; Lorenzo *et al*, 2004).

After the patient leaves the operating suite, the length of hospital stay and any special care involved will contribute a large fraction of the final bill. Procedures that shorten hospital stay are often favored by hospitals, insurers and employers. Some laparoscopic techniques, such as laparoscopic hysterectomy, have only proven their economic worth through shorter recovery times, and thus are most advantageous when applied to members of the working public (Lenihan *et al*, 2004).

The overall cost of a procedure includes the price of convalescence, follow-up and potential morbidity. The cost incurred by society is difficult to measure as this encompasses the most difficult-to-measure variables such as the economic impact of time away from gainful employment and the impact on healthcare resources. The piece of this whole that often leaves the deepest scar is the cost to the healthcare institution providing the services. When reimbursement does not cover costs, hospitals take a loss. One study in Sweden found that while the burden on society was no greater after laparoscopic colon resection, the healthcare system clearly paid more (Janson *et al*, 2004). Governments that must make decisions regarding healthcare rationing must weigh societal cost-benefit with the burden felt by the healthcare system.

Measuring the cost of minimally invasive procedures: cost as an outcome

Some of the most important studies comparing laparoscopic and open procedures emerged over the past decade, after laparoscopy had firmly taken hold in many surgical subspecialties. The difficulty in analyzing cost lies in sorting out immeasurable factors such as the long-term costs, and the effect on healthcare systems when patients and referring physicians can choose where to have their surgery. To our knowledge, no one has attempted to quantify or compare the overall cost of laparoscopy to society aside from the data gathered to measure the cost of treating individual disease processes (eg. the cost of treating symptomatic gallstones with laparoscopic versus open cholecystectomy).

Because so much of the cost of a procedure is difficult to quantify, many comparisons of standard and laparoscopic procedures have analyzed only specific components of the overall cost. For example, length of stay or operative time are specific measures that are easily measured and compared. However, a shorter length of stay may be offset by significantly higher operating room costs or the financial burden due to increased risk of complications. *Table 9.1* compares the mean measurable cost (either total hospital charge or adjusted cost) of several laparoscopic procedures with their open counterparts as reported in recent literature. While presented here for illustration purposes, this information represents the respective authors' institutional data, and may not reflect national or international averages.

Table 9.1: Mean cost comparison of selected laparoscopic and open procedures

Procedure	Lap	Open	Reference
Cholecystectomy*	$2808	$3434	Bosch, *et al*
Colectomy for cancer*	Eu 11 660	Eu 9814	Janson, *et al*
Inguinal hernia (extraperitoneal)**	$795	$666	Khajanchee, *et al*
Nephrectomy*	$7468	$8679	Lotan, *et al*
Nissen Fundoplication*	$4807	$9614	Heikkinen, *et al*
Roux-en-Y Gastric Bypass for obesity*	$4180	$3179	Angus, *et al*
Splenectomy for ITP†	$14 310	$11 454	Cordera, *et al*
Vaginal hysterectomy†	$16 459	$6889	Lenihan, *et al*

(*) total hospital cost, (**) direct cost, (†) billed charges, Eu – Euro

Normalizing cost is one way that statisticians can compare procedures, making a ratio of the known costs and benefits (either long or short term). For example, one study from the UK comparing laparoscopic and open inguinal hernia repairs with mesh found that cost-per-recurrence (measurable cost divided by the established effectiveness of the procedure) was higher for the laparoscopic technique, making it a less economically sound choice for repair (Vale *et al*, 2004). When the effectiveness of both laparoscopic and open procedures is comparable, the estimated QALYs (quality adjusted life years) may not reflect a significant benefit despite the short-term benefits of pain and morbidity reduction (Subak and Caughey, 2000).

Tangible outcomes, such as achieving independence from costly medications to treat a condition like gastrosophageal reflux disease, provide a quantifiable saving to the patient and demonstrate one way in which a particular operation (in this case, laparoscopic Nissen fundoplication) can lead to a reduction in healthcare costs (Nessen *et al*, 1999). As another example, diagnostic laparoscopy provides measurable benefit by sometimes obviating the need for an unnecessary, more morbid and costly open procedure. Clinical indecision and the potential complications of serious conditions managed nonoperatively (such as appendicitis, trauma or ruptured tubal pregnancy) may also be avoided when such tools are available (Marks *et al*, 1997; Taner *et al* 2001).

Cost reducing measures aimed at making laparoscopic surgery more affordable include the use of reusable instruments, increasing operating room efficiency in order to reduce operative times, and the development of postoperative clinical pathway guidelines to minimize length of stay (Demoulin *et al*, 1996; Champault *et al*, 2002; Ogan *et al*, 2002; Lotan *et al*, 2002).

Weighing benefit and cost

At times, it is apparent that what insurers and hospitals deem the best approach is not always what the patient or surgeon feels is most appropriate. The primary interest of the healthcare insurer is to make financial ends meet. The hospital must contain costs, but also comply with established ethical and medical standards. The surgeon faces numerous choices and must decide what is best for the patient based on known outcomes data. When given a chance to decide, the patients' concerns are usually less financial and more focused on safety, efficacy and tangible variables like pain and length of convalescence.

The importance of the patient's perspective should never be overlooked. One goal of improvements in surgical outcomes is to benefit the quality of postoperative life (Nguyen *et al*, 2001; Schneider *et al*, 2003; Vale *et al*, 2004). One major way that patient satisfaction can be improved is through reduced post-operative pain, an obvious result of smaller incisions. (Cordera *et al*, 2003) Shorter hospital stays translate into lower nosocomial complications (Dire *et al*, 2003), reduced cost and faster return to gainful employment or schooling (Schneider *et al*, 2003; Lenihan *et al*, 2004), clearly a win-win situation.

Hospital administrators are responsible not only for their patients but for the solvency of their respective institutions. As a result, they have the formidable task of balancing medical necessity with scarce and often expensive resources. Without a clear benefit, either financial or clinical, new technology cannot survive in an environment of cost-containment. An additional issue facing healthcare in the twenty-first century is how small and private hospitals can survive economically and provide state-of-the-art surgical care when larger, academic tertiary care centers draw patients with their greater financial and clinical resources. Finally, one potential benefit of minimally invasive techniques from the hospital's standpoint is the effect on length of stay. Shorter hospitalizations allows for more rapid turnover and greater bed availability (Senagore *et al*, 2002).

Third-party payers must compete for subscribers but have to make far-reaching decisions about what constitutes fair coverage. Turning the rationing of healthcare coverage into a business necessarily generates controversy. Private insurance typically reimburses more for certain laparoscopic operations than public insurance, creating an incentive for surgeons to offer their services more aggressively to privately insured patients (Angus *et al*, 2003).

The priorities of society as a whole favor superior but affordable healthcare. Patient preference is affected by the way new technology is marketed and portrayed. Fear of complications (eg. bleeding, infections) is a powerful motivator of public opinion that must be recognized. The desire of the public to suffer less pain, sustain smaller surgical wounds and recover more quickly generated much of the force that brought laparoscopic surgery into the mainstream.

Surgeons and physicians, seek out tools that will be efficacious, safe (Bloom *et al*, 1973) and relatively easy to use. In addition, to survive in a competitive environment and build a practice, both cost and marketability become at least secondary issues. Primary care physicians base their referral patterns at least partially on the skill and success of a surgeon. As a result of these factors, new technology such as laparoscopy and minimally invasive techniques in general are sought by patients and provided by surgeons, but should be critically evaluated for safety and efficacy (Hopkins, 2000).

Conclusions

Minimally invasive surgery is here to stay. Each year, new techniques stemming from the desire to reduce the morbidity of surgery are being developed and should be closely appraised by surgeons for safety and applicability. As a relatively new branch of medical technology, laparoscopy provides clear benefits and alternatives for surgeons and their patients, but as with all new developments, it comes with a cost.

In order to become economically acceptable, laparoscopic and other minimally invasive procedures must offset the greater equipment and overhead costs with shorter lengths of stay and shorter operating times. The obvious benefit to the patient (ie, reduced morbidity and discomfort postoperatively) comprises the primary drive to develop new, minimally invasive surgical technology and make it available to the public.

Key points for *Chapter 9*

- Providers and consumers must function in an environment of cost-containment where cost is increasingly seen as a measurable outcome of medical treatment.

- The safety, clinical utility, effectiveness and cost of any new technology should be critically analyzed.

- Reduced morbidity and shorter recovery time both lead to improved productivity, a component of cost that is difficult to quantify.

- Minimally invasive procedures are typically less painful and more cosmetically satisfying, benefits that may outweigh greater medical expense in a consumer-driven market.

- Society must weigh the availability of new technology and the preferences of the patient against limited healthcare resources.

References

Angus LD, Cottam DR *et al* (2003) DRG, costs and reimbursement following Roux-en-Y gastric bypass: an economic appraisal. *Obes Surg* **13(4):** 591–5

Bloom BS, Goldhaber SZ *et al* (1973) Fiberoptics: morbidity and cost. *N Engl J Med* **288(7):** 368–9

Bosch F, Wehrman U *et al* (2002) Laparoscopic or open conventional cholecystectomy: clinical and economic considerations. *Eur J Surg* **168(5):** 270–7

Champault A, Vons C *et al* (2002) Low-cost laparoscopic cholecystectomy. *Br J Surg* **89(12):** 1602–7

Cordera F, Long KH *et al* (2003) Open versus laparoscopic splenectomy for idiopathic thrombocytopenic purpura: clinical and economic analysis. *Surgery* **134(1):** 45–52

Demoulin L, Kesteloot K *et al* (1996) A cost comparison of disposable *vs.* reusable instruments in laparoscopic cholecystectomy. *Surg Endosc* **10(5):** 520–5

Dire CA, Jones MP *et al* (2003) The economics of laparoscopic Nissen fundoplication. *Clin Gastroenterol Hepatol* **1(4):** 328–32

Ferreira MR, Bennett RL *et al* (1999) Diffusion of Laparoscopic Cholecystectomy in the Veterans Affairs Health Care System, 1991–1995. *Eff Clin Pract* **2(2):** 49–55

Heikkinen TJ, Haukipuro K *et al* (1999) Comparison of costs between laparoscopic and open Nissen fundoplication: a prospective randomized study with a 3-month follow-up. *J Am Coll Surg* **188(4):** 368–76

Hopkins MP (2000) The myths of laparoscopic surgery. *Am J Obstet Gynecol* **183(1):** 1–5

Janson M, Bjorholt I *et al* (2004) Randomized clinical trial of the costs of open and laparoscopic surgery for colonic cancer. *Br J Surg* **91(4):** 409–17

Khajanchee YS, Kenyon TA *et al* (2004). Economic evaluation of laparoscopic and open inguinal herniorrhaphies: the effect of cost-containment measures and internal hospital policy decisions on costs and charges. *Hernia* **8(3):** 196–202

Lenihan JP Jr, Kovanda C *et al* (2004) Comparison of laparoscopic-assisted vaginal hysterectomy with traditional hysterectomy for cost-effectiveness to employers. *Am J Obstet Gynecol* **190(6):**1714–20; discussion 1720–2

Link RE, Su LM *et al* (2004) Making ends meet: a cost comparison of laparoscopic and open radical retropubic prostatectomy. *J Urol* **172(1):** 269–74

Lorenzo AJ, Samuelson ML *et al* (2004) Cost analysis of laparoscopic versus open orchiopexy in the management of unilateral nonpalpable testicles. *J Urol* **172(2):** 712–6

Lotan Y, Gettman MT *et al* (2002) Cost comparison for laparoscopic nephrectomy and open nephrectomy: analysis of individual parameters. *Urology* **59(6):** 821–5

Marks JM, Youngelman DF *et al* (1997) Cost analysis of diagnostic laparoscopy *vs.* laparotomy in the evaluation of penetrating abdominal trauma. *Surg Endosc* **11(3):** 272–6

Mouret, P (1990) Celioscopic surgery. Evolution or Revolution? *Chirurgie* **116(10):** 829–32

Nenner RP, Imperato PJ *et al* (1994) Increased cholecystectomy rates among Medicare patients after the introduction of laparoscopic cholecystectomy. *J Community Health* **19:** 409–15

Nessen SC, Holcomb J *et al* (1999) Early laparoscopic Nissen fundoplication for recurrent reflux esophagitis: a cost-effective alternative to omeprazole. *JSLS* **3(2):** 103–6

Nguyen NT, Goldman C *et al* (2001) Laparoscopic versus open gastric bypass: a randomized study of outcomes, quality of life, and costs. *Ann Surg* **234(3):** 279–89; discussion 289–91

Ogan K, Lotan Y *et al* (2002) Laparoscopic versus open retroperitoneal lymph node dissection: a cost analysis. *J Urol* **168(5):** 1945–9; discussion 1949

Schneider BE, Castillo JM *et al* (2003) Laparoscopic totally extraperitoneal versus Lichtenstein herniorrhaphy: cost comparison at teaching hospitals. *Surg Laparosc Endosc Percutan Tech* **13(4):** 261–7

Senagore AJ, Duepree HJ *et al* (2002) Cost structure of laparoscopic and open sigmoid colectomy for diverticular disease: similarities and differences. *Dis Colon Rectum* **45(4):** 485–90

Subak LL, Caughey AB (2000) Measuring cost-effectiveness of surgical procedures. *Clin Obstet Gynecol* **43(3):** 551–60

Taner AS, Topgul K *et al* (2001) Diagnostic laparoscopy decreases the rate of unnecessary laparotomies and reduces hospital costs in trauma patients. *J Laparoendosc Adv Surg Tech A* **11(4):** 207–11

Vale L, Grant A *et al* (2004) EU Hernia Trialists Collaboration. Cost-effectiveness of alternative methods of surgical repair of inguinal hernia. *Int J Technol Assess Health Care* **20(2):** 192–200

Wheeless CR Jr (1976) Laparoscopy. *Clin Obstet Gynecol* **19(2):** 277–98

CHAPTER 10

Impact of laparoscopy on organ donation: living donor nephrectomy

A Alcaraz, HRH Patel

Advances in transplantation science are helping to save more lives than ever, however, there is a critical shortage of organ donations and a continually growing list of patients waiting for a life saving transplant. The arrival of Laparoscopic Living Donor Nephrectomy (LLDN) in the last decade has increased worldwide the availability of organs for donor transplants. Currently, approximately half of the kidney transplants in the US and around 10% in Europe are living donor.

Introduction

Advances in transplantation science are helping to save more lives than ever (Wolfe *et al*, 1999). However, there is a critical shortage of organ donations and a continually growing list of patients waiting for a life saving transplant. This makes organ sharing a very topical issue, which has caused a great deal of ethical debate.

To overcome the lack of cadaveric organs, living donor supply has become the preferred procedure in the US, while expanding criteria for cadaveric donors, including aging and non-heart-beating donors, is the most common in Europe. The arrival of Laparoscopic Living Donor Nephrectomy (LLDN) in the last decade has increased worldwide the trend to perform more living donors than cadaveric donor transplants. Currently, approximately half of the kidney transplants in the US and around 10% in Europe are living donor.

This chapter reviews the impact of the laparoscopic procedure on the number of kidney transplants; a debate between advantages and potential disadvantages of living donor over cadaveric donor and laparoscopic organ retrieval over the open procedure.

Impact on number of transplants

US kidney transplantations

To date, more than 300000 transplants for all organs in the United States. Approximately 20% of these are living donation. In 2003, however, approximately half of kidney transplants came from living donors (*Figure 10.1*).

The number of cadaveric donor kidneys transplanted has remained static at less than 7000 per year, including about 850 (12%) from expanded criteria. The number of living donor kidney transplants reported to the OPTN/UNOS (Organ Procurement and Transplant Network/United Network for Organ Sharing) registry more than doubled during the decade from 1992–2002, from 2535 to 6236, with the largest increases in transplants from offspring to their parents and from spouses and other genetically unrelated donors (*Figure 10.1*; Cecka, 2003).

Since its first description in 1995, laparoscopic live donor nephrectomy has replaced open nephrectomy over a relatively short time span at many transplant centers (2001 Annual Report, 2002). Some investigators have even suggested that the availability of the minimally invasive procurement mode has significantly contributed to the recent increase of live kidney donations in the United States (5-6) (Flowers *et al*, 1997; Schweitzer *et al*, 2000).

From 1 November, 1999 to 21 December, 2000, the number of UNOS-accredited kidney transplant programs reporting laparoscopic nephrectomies increased from fifty-eight (30% of all kidney programs) to eighty (41% of all kidney programs). Similarly, the proportion of laparoscopic kidney grafts increased from 34.9% in November 1999 to 53.5% in December 2000, while the proportion of open kidney graft diminished from 51.1% to 35.0%, respectively. During the study period (Cecka, 2003), 6073 live donor kidney transplants were reported to UNOS. Of the 6073 kidney procurements from live donors, 2734 (45%) were carried out with a laparoscopic approach, 2953 (48.6%) with an open approach. In 386 (6.4%) cases, the procurement technique had not been reported.

Spain has the highest cadaveric kidney donation rate in the world (34.6 donors per million inhabitants) resulting in 49.2 cadaveric kidney transplants per million inhabitants (2125 during the year 2004) (*Figure 10.2*). Despite this high donation rate, waiting lists remain stable around 4000 patients. Until 2002 kidney transplants from living donors represented less

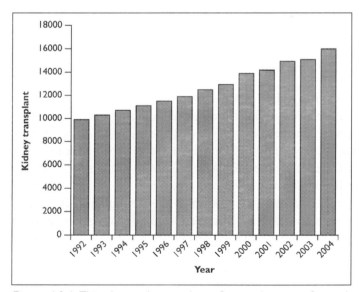

Figure 10.1: This shows the number of transplants performed each year from 1992 to 2004 in the USA (Fehrman-Ekholm et al, 2001; Cecka, 2003). Of note the progressive increase of the number of transplants.

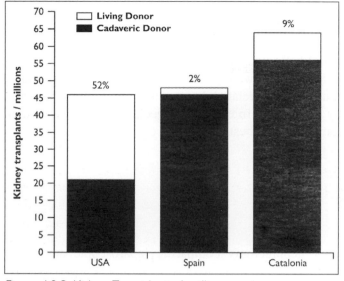

Figure 10.2: Kidney Transplants / million

than 1% of the total. Currently, two out of six transplant centers in Catalonia have begun their laparoscopic living donor programs (the only ones in Spain) resulting in a 9% rate of living donor kidney transplant. (International figures on organ donation, 2004)

Together, laparoscopy and the improvement in the management of acute rejection are responsible for increasing the number of living donor transplants. As kidney transplantation has progressed and antirejection drugs have improved, an increasing number of organs have come from living donors. It is now common for transplant patients to receive a kidney from a family member or friend. Despite the rise in more HLA-incompatible living donors, five year graft survival rates among recipients transplanted between 1998 and 2002 were 78.5% and 77.5% for spouse and other unrelated donor grafts, respectively, and were comparable to that for one-haplotype-matched sibling transplant (80.7%). As already said, in recent years, more patients have received living-donor kidney transplants in the US than cadaveric kidney transplants. This is the first time this has happened since the earliest days of kidney transplantation, when only the identical twin of a recipient could donate a kidney.

Living donor advantages

Living-donor kidney transplantation has some advantages over cadaveric kidney transplantation. Moreover, waiting time on dialysis has been associated with worse outcomes after living and cadaveric transplantation (Meier-Krische and Kaplan, 2002). Once a living donor has been found, the operation can be scheduled at the donor and recipient's convenience.

Many recipients are already on the waiting list for a cadaveric kidney. Those who receive living-donor kidney transplants often spend significantly less time on the list than cadaveric kidney recipients. A living-donor operation can often be performed within three months of identifying a donor. More than 60% of living-donor kidney recipients were transplanted within two years of starting dialysis, compared with fewer than 20% of those who received a cadaveric donor kidney. The average wait for a cadaveric kidney ranges from two to six years – depending on blood type, cross-matching, and a variety of other factors.

In the above mentioned report, data available from the US Renal Data System database between 1988 and 1998 were analyzed to quantify the effect of end stage renal disease (ESRD), time on paired cadaveric kidneys and on all cadaveric kidneys compared to living-donated kidneys. It was proved that ESRD time was the strongest independent modifiable risk factor for renal transplant outcomes. Part of the advantage of living-donor versus cadaveric-donor transplantation may be explained by waiting time (Meier-Krische and Kaplan, 2002). This effect is dominant enough that a cadaveric renal transplant recipient with an ESRD time less than six months has the equivalent graft survival of living donor transplant recipients who wait on dialysis for more than two years.

Outcomes after kidney transplantation using living-related donors have always been superior to those using cadaveric donors, especially in the modern era of antirejection therapy. In certain types of patients, such as infants, living donation is the best option.

Laparoscopic LDN advantages

Several systematic reviews of living-donor nephrectomy comparing laparoscopic and open procedure have been published (Troppmann *et al*, 2003). In the review of 687 publications, twenty studies with level I-II evidence and twelve with level III evidence were analyzed. Only one level I study could be identified. Level I and level II evidence suggest superiority of the laparoscopic approach in regard to postoperative analgesic consumption, hospital stay and return to work. Other safety and efficacy criteria, including donor and recipient outcomes, were similar between the two techniques. A review by Matas *et al* (Matas *et al*, 2003) stresses the doubt about safety in the laparoscopic procedures.

Multiple studies have shown that laparoscopic nephrectomy is considerably gentler for the donor, because it is associated with less postoperative pain, a shorter length of hospital stay, improved cosmesis, and faster return to work and activities of daily living.

Potential laparoscopic LDN disadvantages

Laparoscopic nephrectomy has undeniable benefits for the donor; however, the implications of this new surgical technique for the recipient have been controversial for at least three reasons. First, initial reports suggested higher vascular and ureteral complication rates with laparoscopically procured kidney grafts. However, subsequent studies have demonstrated that with increasing surgical experience, low technical complication rates can also be achieved with laparoscopic kidneys, regardless of whether left or right kidneys (Lind *et al*, 2002), or kidneys with anatomical variations, such as multiple renal arteries, are used (Alcaraz *et al*, 2005).

Second, several investigators have shown slower early post-transplant function for laparoscopic grafts, as measured by delayed function rates and by the recipient's early post-transplant serum creatinine levels. These findings are not surprising, because warm ischemia times in laparoscopic donors are longer; and the pneumoperitoneum created during the laparoscopic operation negatively affects renal hemodynamics.

Slower early function in laparoscopic grafts, however, was not observed on all post-transplant days, did not persist beyond the first month, and did not achieve statistical significance at all time points in all studies. Also, other reports have suggested equivalent early graft function after laparoscopic and open kidney procurement (Wolf *et al*, 1998; Stifelman *et al*, 2001). In our experience (Alcaraz *et al*, 2004) we could achieve the creatinine nadir on the second day after transplantation (126 μmol/ml), with no differences with the open series.

Since warm ischemia time does not appear to be the determining factor in delayed graft function, intraoperative renal perfusion seems important and several measures should be taken. Hydration with intravenous fluids and osmotic diuretics should be used to ameliorate the negative effect of peritoneal cavity insufflation which causes a reflex decrease in urine output, possibly resulting from renal venous outflow compression. Renal arterial traction should be avoided during dissection because it may lead to decreased perfusion due to vasospasm or intimal injury. Papaverine can be used in order to avoid arterial vasospasm. Compressing the renal parenchyma during organ extraction may cause parenchymal edema with subsequent decreased tissue perfusion.

Third, and the major disadvantage is the risk for the living donor, including perioperative morbidity and mortality, plus the long term risk of living with a single kidney. Morbidity and mortality (0.03%) after open nephrectomy were described decades ago (Najarian *et al*, 1992; Bia *et al*, 1995). Mortality rates remain unchanged even after the introduction of laparoscopic nephrectomy (0.03%). The three deaths reported to UNOS may be due to a lack of experience (Matas *et al*, 2003). Life threatening complications, mainly due to vascular injury during dissection, are the most common cause of conversion to open surgery (2% in very experienced series) (Jacobs *et al*, 2004) and reoperation (1%) (Matas *et al*, 2003). To minimize the effect of these complications, avoiding potentially catastrophic outcomes, after finalizing the laparoscopic dissection of the kidney we perform a hand-extraction of the kidney that allows us a gentle traction of the kidney resulting in good vessel length, as well as an immediate control if necessary of pedicle bleeding.

The risks of living with a single kidney include the possible long-term adverse effect on the renal function and blood pressure of the donors. Fehrman-Ekholm *et al* (Fehrman-Ekholm *et al*, 2001) can clarify this issue since it is able to overpass the low donor-participation rate, the major weakness in almost all of the follow-up reported studies. They performed a comprehensive follow-up of all living kidney donors at their center from 1964 to 1995. Of 402 donors still alive, they were able to get information about serum creatinine, urinary proteins, and blood cells in urine using reagent trips, and blood pressure from 87% of them. In the study, none of the donors had died of end-stage renal disease (ESRD). On average, the remaining renal function of kidney donors did not deteriorate more rapidly than what may be expected from ageing, and the prevalence of hypertension is not increased compared with age-matched controls. This study supports the continued use of living kidney donors, using a strict criteria guideline.

Ethical and moral considerations

Altruistic donation between spouses and other genetically unrelated people is currently fully accepted as commercial transplant is fully refused. Traditionally, medical associations and human rights groups around the world have condemned the buying and selling of human organs. The World Health Organisation (WHO) (WHO, 1991) declares the commercialization of human organs to be 'a violation of human rights' and 'human dignity'. In its 1991 document 'Guiding Principles on Human Organ Transplantation', the WHO expresses concern over 'the rise of commercial traffic in human organs, particularly from living donors who are unrelated to recipients'. It lays down this guiding principle: 'The human body and its parts cannot be the subject of commercial transactions. Accordingly, giving or receiving payment (including any other compensation or reward) for organs should be prohibited'.

Over the past two decades, the Transplantation Society, through its Ethics Committee, has consistently opposed paid organ donation, its position being: 'organs and tissues should be freely given without commercial or financial profit'. The American Society of Transplant Surgeons and professional association in Europe, Canada and Britain have also condemned the organ trade. This is at one level. However, with demand for healthy kidneys for transplantation far outstripping supply, international debate has occurred on whether traditional ethical and moral values should be put aside and the sale of organs legalized. It is argued that society has a collective responsibility to save lives and therefore must set aside ethical notions such as altruism and the inviolability of the human body.

Proponents of paid donor schemes argue for a regulated market in kidneys such as the system adopted by Iran in 1997. Such a market will be self-regulating. Rising demand will raise the price of organs in short supply, creating incentives for people to sell their kidneys. This in turn will ensure that enough organs are available to meet the demand.

Conclusions

Laparoscopic donor nephrectomy has gained community acceptance by physicians and patients over the past decade. Despite a lack of strong evidence, such as large prospective randomized studies, this change in practice was mostly driven by the donors needs and expectations. However, laparoscopic donor nephrectomy has been proven to be superior to open nephrectomy in terms of postoperative pain, early recovery and improved cosmesis, maintaining the standards of safety and efficacy. Laparoscopic donor nephrectomy is likely to become the gold standard for donor nephrectomy in the near future.

Key points for *Chapter 10*

- The arrival of Laparoscopic Living Donor Nephrectomy (LLDN) in the last decade has increased worldwide the availability of organs for donor transplants.
- Approximately half of the kidney transplants in the US and around 10% in Europe are living donor.
- Advances in transplantation science are helping to save more lives than ever before.
- Since its first description in 1995, laparoscopic live donor nephrectomy has replaced open nephrectomy over a relatively short time span at many transplant centers.
- To date, there have been more than 300000 transplants for all organs in the United States.
- The number of living donor kidney transplants reported to the OPTN/UNOS registry more than doubled during the decade from 1992–2002, from 2535 to 6236, with the largest increases in transplants from offspring to their parents and from spouses and other genetically unrelated donors.
- Laparoscopic donor nephrectomy has been proven to be superior to open nephrectomy in terms of postoperative pain, early recovery and improved cosmesis, maintaining the standards of safety and efficacy.
- Laparoscopic donor nephrectomy is likely to become the 'gold standard' for donor nephrectomy in the near future.
- Laparoscopic donor nephrectomy will help to decrease the illegal trade in organ 'donation'.

References

Alcaraz A, Rosales A *et al* (2004) Laparoscopic nephrectomy in living donor for renal transplant. Experience of two years. *Arch Esp Urol* **57:** 10

Alcaraz A, Rosales A *et al* (2005) Multiple artery pedicle in living donor kidney transplant. Transplant Proceed (in press)

Bia MJ, Ramos EL *et al* (1995) Evaluation of living renal donors. The current practice of US transplant center. *Transplantation* **60:** 322–7

Cecka JM. The OPTN/UNOS Renal Transplant Registry 2003. *Clinic Transp* 1–12

Fehrman-Ekholm I, Duner F *et al* (2001) No evidence of accelerated loss of kidney function in living kidney donors: results from a cross-sectional follow-up. *Transplantation* 15; **72:** 444–9

Flowers JL, Jacobs S *et al* (1997) Comparison of open and laparoscopic live donor nephrectomy. *Ann Surg* **226:** 483–189

International figures on organ donation and transplantation year 2003 (2004) *Newsletter Transplant* **9(1):** 5–17

Jacobs S, Cho E *et al* (2004) Laparoscopic donor nephrectomy: the University of Maryland 6-year experience. *J Urol* **171:** 47–51

Lind MY, Hazebroek EJ *et al* (2002) Right-sided laparoscopic live-donor nephrectomy: is reluctance still justified? *Transplantation* **74(15):** 1045–8

Matas AJ, Bartlett ST *et al* (2003) Morbidity and mortality after living kidney donation, 1999–2001: survey of United States Transplant Centers. *Am J of Transplant* **7:** 830

Meier-Krische HU, Kaplan B (2002) Waiting time on dialysis as the strongest modifiable risk factor for renal transplant outcomes: a paired donor kidney analysis. *Transplantation* **74:** 1377–81

Najarian JS, Chavero BM *et al* (1992) 20 years or more of follow-up of living kidney donors. *Lancet* **340(8823):** 807–10

Schweitzer EJ, Wilson J *et al* (2000) Increased rates of donation with laparoscopic donor nephrectomy. *Ann Surg* **232:** 392–400

Stifelman MD, Hull D *et al* (2001) Hand assisted laparoscopic donor nephrectomy: a comparison with the open approach. *J Urol* **166(2):** 444–8

Troppmann C, Ormond DB *et al* (2003) Laparoscopic (*vs.* Open) live donor nephrectomy: a UNOS database analysis of early graft function and survival. *Am J of Transplant* **3:** 1295–1301

UNOS (2001) Annual Report (2002) Vol. 1. United Network for Organ Sharing Richmond, VA 32

WHO (1991) Resolution WHA44.25 on *Guiding principles on human organ transplantation. Adopted by the 50% (more than what is found in the majority of 44th WH Assembly.* WHO, Geneva

Wolf JS, Tchetgen MB *et al* (1998) Hand-assisted laparoscopic live donor nephrectomy. *Urology* **52:** 885

Wolfe RA, Ashby VB *et al* (1999) Comparison of mortality in all patients on dialysis, patients on dialysis awaiting transplantation, and recipients of a first cadaveric transplant. *N Engl J Med.* **341:** 1725

CHAPTER 11

Minimal access surgery in urogynecology

R Kearney, A Cutner

Operations for stress urinary incontinence and pelvic organ prolapse are frequently performed and in recent years the range of minimally invasive procedures available for the treatment of these problems has expanded.

Stress incontinence can be managed by laparoscopic colposuspension or by the placement of a synthetic suburethral sling. The only synthetic sling subjected to randomised control trial is the Tension free Vaginal Tape (TVT) (Gynecare). This has been shown to produce a similar cure rate to open colposuspension in women undergoing surgery for primary stress urinary incontinence. Injectable therapy is associated with short term improvement in incontinence.

Prolapse of the vaginal vault can be managed surgically by sacrospinous fixation, laparoscopic sacrocolpopexy or the newer posterior intravaginal slingplasty. There are no trials comparing the laparoscopic sacrocoplopexy to the open approach and there is very little data on the efficacy of the posterior intravaginal slingplasty.

There is now a wide selection of minimally invasive procedures available for the treatment of incontinence and prolapse. However there is little outcome data to support the use of some of these procedures and caution must be exercised until there is further information available as to their safety and long term efficacy.

Introduction

The surgical management of pelvic floor dysfunction is rapidly changing with 11% of women seeking surgery to cure the debilitating problems of stress urinary incontinence and pelvic organ prolapse (Olsen *et al*, 1997). Currently there are a myriad of surgical treatments available with new techniques and devices emerging every year. A lot of these techniques are minimally invasive compared with the more traditional operations. This chapter will briefly discuss some of the more widely used minimally invasive techniques and the current knowledge regarding their safety and efficacy. The specific operative techniques will not be discussed in detail as this is beyond the scope of this chapter.

Minimal access surgery for stress urinary incontinence

Laparoscopic colposuspension

The term laparoscopic colposuspension is currently used to describe several different surgical procedures requiring varying levels of laparoscopic surgical skill and with different success rates. The previously considered gold standard operation for stress incontinence was the Tanagho method of a Burch Colposuspension (Tanagho, 1976). This same operation can be performed laparoscopically differing only in the mode of access to the Cave of Retzius. This was first described by Liu in 1993 (Liu and Paek, 1993). Vancaille and Schuessler described a laparoscopic modification of the Marshall Marchetti Kranz procedure in 1991 (Marshall *et al*, 1949; Vancaile and Schuessler, 1991). Subsequent to this many other methods of elevating the vagina have been reported including using mesh and tacs, staples, glue and bipolar electrochemical energy (Ou *et al*, 1993; Kiilholma *et al*, 1995; Birken and Leggett, 1997; Ross *et al*, 2002). The method we favour is a transperitoneal laparoscopic Burch colposuspension using two non-absorbable 0 Ethibond® sutures to elevate the vagina (*Figure 11.1*).

The data comparing laparoscopic colposuspension to the traditional open colposuspension are difficult to interpret due to the variations in techniques described and the methodology of the studies.

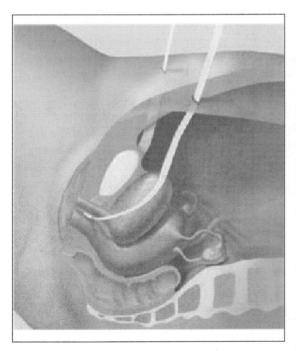

Figure 11.1: The image on the left shows the placement of two sutures on either side at laparoscopic colposuspension. The image on the right demonstrates shortening of the uterosacral ligaments for the treatment of uterine prolapse

The Cochrane database in 2002 concluded that the performance of laparoscopic colposuspension is still uncertain (Moehrer *et al*, 2002). There are four randomized trials which compare the laparoscopic and open approaches using sutures in both arms (Su *et al*, 1997; Burton, 1997; Fatthy *et al*, 2001; Cheon *et al*, 2003). In one of these trials the randomisation was flawed as patients who decided not to proceed with the laparoscopic route after randomization were included in the open group (Su *et al*, 1997). This study reported a lower success rate at one year in the laparoscopic arm (80.4% *vs*. 95.6%). One study performed early in the learning curve of the primary surgeon with absorbable sutures showed a lower cure rate at one year in the laparoscopic arm (60% *vs*. 93%) (Burton, 1997). The two remaining studies showed similar cure rates at one year in the open and laparoscopic arms (85 *vs*. 87.9%, 86 *vs*. 85%) (Fatthy *et al*, 2001; Cheon *et al*, 2003). The laparoscopic procedure is associated with less blood loss and shorter recovery (Su *et al*, 1997; Fatthy *et al*, 2001). One study has shown that using two sutures each taking a single bite of vagina is more effective than one suture taking a double bite (83 *vs*. 58%) (Persson and Wolner-Hanssen, 2000). Interestingly in the Su study only one suture was used in the laparoscopic arm (Su *et al*, 1997).

The most commonly used modification reported as a laparoscopic coplosuspension is the use of mesh and tacs or staples. This involves inserting one or two pieces of prolene mesh lengthwise along the paravaginal fascia at the bladder neck and attaching it to Cooper's ligament with tacs or staples. It is the difficulty in learning suturing techniques that has resulted in the introduction of this and other methods of elevating the vagina. One randomized trial comparing laparoscopic colposuspension using mesh and tacs with sutures showed a higher failure rate at one year with the mesh technique (26.9 *vs*. 11.1%). (Zullo *et al*, 2001)

In a review of 1867 patients the overall complication rate of laparoscopic colposuspension was reported as 10.3% (Buller and Cundif, 2000). The lower urinary tract is injured in 2–3% of cases which is much lower than the 10% reported with the open procedure (Stevenson *et al*, 1999; Miklos and Kohli, 2000; Speights *et al*, 2000). With the use of mesh and tacs other complications have been found including tacs in the bladder (Kenton *et al*, 2002).

Suburethral slings

The concept of using a mid urethral tape to surgically treat stress urinary incontinence was first proposed by Ulmsten in 1996 based on the integral theory of incontinence (Petros and Ulmsten, 1990). Since the advent of the first commercially available tension free vaginal tape (TVT Gynecare), there are now more than fifteen midurethral tapes marketed for the treatment of stress incontinence. Most of the commercially available suburethral synthetic tapes are polypropylene tapes as woven monofilaments (TVT, SPARC, Monarc, Uretex Sup, Advantage), multi-filaments (Intravaginal slingplasty (IVs), SAFYRE comprising two silicone tension bands), extruded crosslinked polypropylene (Obtape) or silicone-coated polypropylene in contact with the urethra (Uratape).

There are four methods of insertion in current use. Ulmsten described insertion of a suburethral tape as a day procedure under local anesthetic (Ulmsten *et al*, 1996). A vertical suburethral incision is made in the vagina and after dissecting towards the retopubic space on either side of the urethra, the tape is introduced with a trocar and tunneller traversing the retropubic space to emerge suprapubically. Ulmsten reported a 84% cure rate at two years. By 2001 over 100000 TVT procedures had been performed (Ulmsten *et al*, 2001). The TVT (Gynecare, Johnson&Johnson) is made of monofilament polypropylene and has been the most extensively evaluated tape in research studies. Indeed many of the more recent commercially available tapes have become available for clinical use with little prior scientific evidence as to their safety and efficacy. The IVs tunneller (TYCO) has a blunt tip compared to the sharp tip of the TVT trocar. The tape is a knitted polypropylene polymer. It can be used vaginally or abdominally. There is little data available on its efficacy. The Advantage mesh (Boston Scientific) is also a monofilament polypropylene mesh with a de-tangled portion in the suburethral portion

Following the vaginal approach being established, a suprapubic approach was developed. The trocar was inserted from the suprapubic region downwards to emerge in the vaginal incision. The SPARC tape (AMS) was designed to be inserted from the top down. The tape is inserted using needles that are thinner than the other trocars on the market and the tape has a tensioning suture to stop fraying. A trial of 104 women reported an objective cure rate of 90% and a subjective cure rate of 72% (Deval *et al*, 2003). One study comparing it with TVT has shown that the placement of the SPARC is more cranial, further away from the symphysis pubis and more mobile than the TVT (Dietz *et al*, 2004). Bioarc (AMS) is similar to the SPARC but is designed to allow placement of a biologic suburethral implant. Lynx (Boston Scientific) is another suprapubic midurethral sling using the same mesh as Advantage.

Uretex (Bard) is a knitted polypropylene mesh that can be inserted suprapubically or vaginally. SAFYRE (Promedon) is marketed as a self-anchoring readjustable sling after surgery. The polypropylene mesh is anchored between two columns of silicone and is inserted with a needle that can be used transvaginally or suprapubically. A prospective non randomized clinical study of 126 women reported a 92% continent rate at eighteen months. The tape was loosened postoperatively in 3% of women and tightened in 5% (Palma *et al*, 2005). A further 5% of patients presented with vaginal erosion of the tape requiring further surgery.

In 2001 Delorme described the transobturator technique for insertion of a suburethral tape (Delorme, 2001). A similar vaginal incision as the other tapes is used but the tunnel is dissected to the ischiopubic rami on either side. Then an incision is made at the lateral margin of the ischio-pubic ramus on a horizontal line with the clitoris. The tunneller is inserted across the obturator membrane and then turned horizontally to meet a finger in the vaginal incision. The tape (Uratape) is then inserted into the eye of the needle and then the tunneller is withdrawn. Again the tape is tension-free. The advantage of this method is that it avoids major blood vessel, bladder or bowel injury and may be easier in patients who have had previous retropubic surgery than the other methods. Monarc (AMS), Obtryx (Boston Scientific), Mentor (Obtape) are other trans-obturator tapes designed for insertion from outside in. I-STOP (CL medical), Intramesh LIFT (Cousin Biotech), tapes can be used with abdominal, vaginal or via the transobturator approach.

The TVT obturator (Gynecare) is a tape which is placed from inside the vaginal incision to traverse the obturator foramen and emerge lateral to the labia majora.

SABRE is a bioabsorbable sling which is inserted vaginally and PelviLace (Bard) is a porcine acellular collagen matrix sling which can be inserted using the outside in transobturator approach. T-Sling (Caldera Medical) is a polypropylene sling with the option of a polydioxinone bioabsorbable central portion. Stratasis (Cook) is another non-synthetic sling of animal origin. These bioasborbable slings undergo remodelling and may autolyse or become antigenic.

With the exception of TVT there is a paucity of outcome data for the majority of the tapes currently in use. A multicentred randomised trial of TVT and colposuspension has shown equal efficacy between the two procedures at two years (63% *vs.* 51%) (Ward *et al*, 2004). However it must be appreciated that this study assessed the treatment for primary stress incontinence. No additional surgery other than the TVT in one arm and open colposuspension in the other arm was carried out. To translate the findings to patients undergoing concomitant hysterectomy or other prolapse procedures is probably incorrect.

The Cochrane Database for Systemic Reviews of suburethral sling operations for stress incontinence in women states that the success rate of the TVT is similar to that of open retropubic operations but that longer-term data is needed (Bezerra and Bruschini, 2001). The outcome of the TVT is similar if performed under local or spinal anaesthesia (Adamiak *et al*, 2002). Two randomized studies have compared the outcome of TVT with laparoscopic colposuspension (Üstün *et al*, 2003; Valpas *et al*, 2004). One study comparing TVT to the laparoscopic mesh method, demonstrated a higher cure rate at one year in the TVT group (85.7 *vs.* 56.9%) (Valpas *et al*, 2004) The second study used sutures in the laparoscopic arm and reported similar outcomes for both procedures after eighteen months (82%) (Üstün *et al*, 2003).

One retrospective study comparing the TVT and TOT methods showed similar cure rates at eighteen months with a higher rate of bladder injury in the TVT group but a urethral injury occurred in the TOT group (Mellier *et al*, 2004). There is insufficient clinical data on the outcome of the other types of tapes.

Although these procedures are easy to perform there is a risk of injury to the bladder, bowel and major blood vessels with the retropubic tapes (Kobashi and Govier, 2003; Castillo *et al*, 2004; Frankel, 2004). The transobturator tape insertion may also injure the urethra, bladder or the obturator bundle but the overall complication rate reported to date is lower. This is based on very little scientific data and larger long term studies are required to provide more information on the complications of these procedures. Other reported complications include groin pain. All these procedures involve inserting a permanent tape under the urethra, and erosions into the urethra, bladder and vagina and dyspareunia have been reported (Wai *et al*, 2004; McLennan, 2004; Glavind and Sander, 2004; Tsivian *et al*, 2004).

Injectables

The least invasive of surgical treatments for stress incontinence is the use of urethral bulking agents of which there are several currently used. There are variations on the agent used and the method of injection. The first commercially available material for periurethral injection was Teflon. The use of this material has now been abandoned due to problems with erosion, fibrosis and granulomatous reaction (Ferro *et al*, 1988). Next autologous fat was used but this is now rarely used due to the variable success rates (Herschorn, (2001). Currently the most commonly used materials are GAX collagen (Contigen; C. R. Bard) and silicone particles (Macroplastique, Uroplasty). More recently Carbon-coated zirconium beads and a non-animal-stabilized hyaluronic acid /dextranomer (NASHA/Dx) copolymer have been introduced.

Gax Collagen can be introduced either transurethrally or transperineally with a long needle under cystoscopic guidance. All the other substances were introduced using transurethral injection under cystoscopic control. It is felt that the variable success rates may be due to difficulty with accurate placement. Macroplastique then introduced a device for blind injection to make the procedure more standardized and this has been further perfected for the injection of non-animal-stabilised hyaluronic acid /dextranomer (NASHA/Dx) copolymer. Whether these devices improve success rates has yet to be determined. However they do enable the insertion to be under local anesthetic in the outpatient setting.

The main advantages of injectables are the low complication rate and ease of delivery. The Cochrane Database of systemic reviews states that injectable therapy results in a short term improvement and currently they may have a role in women in whom other interventions are unsuitable due to extensive comorbidity precluding anesthesia and surgery (Pickard *et al*, 2003).

Minimal access surgery for pelvic organ prolapse

The surgical management of pelvic organ prolapse continues to be a challenge to the pelvic floor surgeon with 29% of women undergoing surgery requiring a second procedure (Olsen *et al*, 1997). Prolapse may involve the anterior, posterior or central compartments of the pelvic floor. Whatever the type of prolapse it cannot be managed in isolation as the repair of one part of the pelvic floor may impact on the function of other parts. Traditionally the surgical approaches have been either vaginal or open abdominal surgery. However in recent years newer minimally invasive procedures have been introduced. The laparoscopic approach can be used to manage cystocele, rectocele and vault prolapse. The current approaches to the surgical treatment of vault prolapse include sacrospinous fixation, sacrocolpopexy and posterior intravaginal slingplasty.

Laparoscopic paravaginal repair

The aim of paravaginal repair is to restore the lateral attachments of the vaginal wall and the pubocervical fascia to the obturator internus fascia and the arcus tendineus fascia pelvis. The laparoscopic approach provides excellent visualization of the anatomy which is difficult with the open approach and impossible with the vaginal approach. The repair is usually performed with sutures (Miklos and Kohli, 2000). A mesh technique has also been described (Washington and Somers, 2003). The laparoscopic approach has a low complication rate compared with the vaginal approach which is associated with significant complications including ureteric obstruction and a 16% transfusion rate (Young *et al*, 2001, Mallipeddi *et al*, 2001).

Sacrospinous fixation

Sacrospinous fixation is a long established vaginal approach to treating vault prolapse (Nichols, 1982; Carey and Slack, 1994). It involves attaching the vault to the sacrospinous ligament with sutures. Usually the vault is attached in one place to the right ligament although a method of four wall fixation is also described (Morley and DeLancey, 1988). The advantage of the four wall approach is that it allows excision of excess vagina and formation of a new apex to be resuspended (Kearney and DeLancey, 2003). Visualization can be difficult with this operation and complications such as hemorrhage and buttock pain have been reported (Nieminem and Heinonen, 2001; Guner *et al*, 2001). Also anterior compartment prolapse may develop after this procedure (Sze and Karram, 1997).

Laparoscopic sacrocolpopexy

Open sacrocolpopexy involves suspending the vaginal vault to the sacral promontory using a mesh. This was first formally described in 1962 (Lane, 1962). In 1994 a laparoscopic approach was described (Nezhat *et al*, 1994). The ureters are identified and dissected laterally away from the operative area. Then the fascia is opened between the vault and the bladder and the rectum.

A 'y' shaped piece of prolene mesh is placed at the vault and sutured down the anterior and posterior walls and then this is supended to the sacral promontory with tacs. The advantage of the laparoscopic approach is that the mesh can be placed lower down avoiding a vaginal repair of rectocele which would increase the mesh erosion rate.

There are no randomized studies comparing the laparoscopic and open procedures but case series report similar success rates to the open procedure (Mahendran *et al*, 1996: Cosson *et al*, 2000).

The complications of the procedure include bleeding, sacral osteomyelitis and mesh erosion (Weidner *et al*, 1997; Fox and Stanton, 2000; Visco *et al*, 2001).

Posterior intravaginal slingplasty

The posterior intravaginal slingplasty (IV*s*) first described by Petros involves dissecting the vagina at the vault to the ischial spines bilaterally and then inserting a trocar from an incision inferior and lateral to the anus, through the ischiorectal fossa to emerge anterior to the spines. A mesh is then passed through this trocar to emerge out the other side in a similar fashion. This is then attached to the vaginal vault and when the mesh is pulled the vault is elevated. This is a recent procedure and there are very little data on its efficacy. However it is associated with a low morbidity making it a suitable option for medically unfit women (Petros, 200 ; Farnsworth, 2002).

Uterine conserving prolapse surgery

Many women presenting with uterine prolapse request a surgical procedure to alleviate the prolapse while allowing them to conserve their uterus for future fertility. Open sacrohysteropexy has been described with Teflon and Goretex meshes (Constantini *et al*, 1998; Leron and Stanton, 2001). The uterosacral ligaments can be shortened laparoscopically (*Figure 11.1*) (Digesu *et al*, 2004). A laparoscopic suture sacrohysteropexy closing the Pouch of Douglas, shortening the uterosacral ligaments and reattaching them to the cervix has been reported. This has the advantage of quicker recovery and less postoperative adhesions which is important in women considering future fertility (Maher *et al*, 2001). The durability of these procedures unknown but they provide a short term option for women desiring surgical treatment prior to completing their families.

Conclusions

Without doubt the number of surgical procedures that are now available for the treatment of stress urinary incontinence and prolapse is ever expanding. However tempting it is to try the latest technique, it is important that these newer operations are not adopted except in exceptional circumstances outside clinical trials until there are good clinical data to demonstrate their success rates. Too many wonder cures have come and gone in the field of urogynecology in the past.

Key points for *Chapter 11*

■ The lifetime risk of a woman having surgery for incontinence or prolapse is 11% and 29% of these women will require a second procedure.

■ The surgical success of laparoscopic colposuspension for the management of stress urinary incontinence compared with open colposuspension is still uncertain.

■ Laparoscopic colposuspension with sutures is more effective than with mesh and tacs.

■ The TVT procedure is as effective as open colposuspension at two years in women undergoing surgery for primary stress incontinence.

■ There are insufficient data on the long term outcome of the other types of synthetic suburethral slings.

■ The success rate of the obturator tape compared with the retropubic tape is unknown.

■ Suburethral bulking agents result in short term improvement and have the advantage of ease of delivery and a low complication rate.

■ The surgical repair of vaginal vault prolapse can be accomplished laparoscopically or vaginally.

■ The posterior intravaginal slingplasty is a method associated with low morbidity but the long term outcome is unknown.

■ Uterine prolapse in women desiring to conserve their uterus can be managed laparoscopically with good short term results.

References

Adamiak A, Milart P *et al* (2002) The efficacy and safety of the tension-free vaginal tape procedure do not depend on the method of analgesia. *Eur Urol* **4**: 29–33

Bezerra CA, Bruschini H (2001) Suburethral sling operations for urinary incontinence in women. *Cochrane Database Syst Rev* (**3**): CD001754

Birken R, Leggett P (1997) Laparoscopic colposuspension using mesh reinforcement. *Surg Endosc* **11**: 1111–4

Buller J and Cundiff G (2000) Laparoscopic surgeries for urinary incontinence. *Clin Obstet Gynecol* **43**: 604–18

Burton G (1997) A three year prospective randomized urodynamic study comparing open and laparascopic colposuspension. *Neurourol Urodyn* **16**: 353–4

Carey M, Slack M (1994) Vaginal vault prolapse. *Br J Hosp Med* **51**: 417–20

Castillo OA, Bodden E *et al* (2004) Intestinal perforation: an infrequent complication during insertion of tension-free vaginal tape. *J Urol*: 1721364

Cheon W, Mak J *et al* (2003) Prospective randomised controlled trial comparing laparoscopic and open colposuspension. *Hong Kong Med J* **9:** 10–4

Constantini E, Lombi R *et al* (1998) Colposacropexy with Gore-tex mesh in marked vaginal and uterovaginal prolapse. *Eur Urol* **34:** 11–7

Cosson M, Bogaert E *et al* (2000) Laparoscopic sacral colpopexy: short-term results and complications in 83 patients. *J Gynecol Obstet Biol Reproduct* (Paris) **29:** 746–50

Delorme E (2001) Transobturator urethral suspension: mini-invasive procedure in the treatment of stress urinary incontinence in women *Prog Urol* **11:** 1306–13

Deval B, Levardon M *et al* (2003) A French multicenter clinical trial of SPARC for stress urinary incontinence. *Eur Urol* **44(2):** 254–8

Dietz HP, Foote AJ *et al* (2004) TVT and Sparc suburethral slings: a case-control series. *Int Urogynecol J Pelvic Floor Dysfunct* **15(2):** 129–31

Digesu G, Khullar V *et al* (2004) A case of laparoscopic uterosacral ligaments placation: a newconservative approach to uterine prolapse? *Eur J Obstet Gynecol Reprod Biol* **114:** 112–5

Duckett JR, Jain S (2005) Groin pain after a tension-free vaginal tape or similar suburethral sling: management strategies. *Brit J Urol Int* **95:** 95–7

Farnsworth BN (2002) Posterior intravaginal slingplasty (infracoccygeal sacropexy) for severe posthysterectomy vaginal vault prolapse-a preliminary report on efficacy and safety. *Int Urogynecol J Pelvic Floor Dysfunct* **13:** 4–8

Fatthy H, El Hao M *et al* (2001) Modified Burch colposuspension: Laparoscopy versus laparotomy. *J Amer Assoc Gynecol Laparosc* **8:** 99–106

Ferro M, Smith J *et al* (1988) Periurethral granuloma: unusual complication of Teflon periurethral injection. *Urology* **31:** 422–3

Fox S, Stanton S (2000) Vault prolapse and rectocoele: assessment of repair using sacrocolpopexy with mesh interposition. *Brit J Obstet Gynaecol* **107:** 1371–5

Frankel G (2004) Re: Complication of bowel perforation during insertion of tension-free vaginal tape. *J Urol* **171:** 1888

Glavind K, Sander P (2004) Erosion, defective healing and extrusion after tension-free urethropexy for the treatment of stress urinary incontinence. *Int Urogynecol J Pelvic Floor Dysfunct* **15:** 179–82

Guner H, Noyan V *et al* (2001) Transvaginal sacrospinous colpoexy for marked uterovaginal and vault prolapse. *Int J Gynaecol Obstet* **74:** 165–70

Herschorn S (2001) Current status of injectable agents for female stress urinary incontinence. *Can J Urol* **8:** 1281

Kearney R, DeLancey J (2003) Selecting suspension points and excising the vagina during Michigan four wall sacrospinous fixation. *Obstet Gynecol* **101:** 325–30

Kenton K, FitzGerald MP *et al* (2002) Multiple foreign body erosions after laparoscopic colposuspension with mesh. *Am J Obstet Gynecol* **187:** 252–3

Kiilholma P, Haarala M *et al* (1995) Sutureless colposuspension with fibrin sealant. *Tech Urol* **1:** 81–3

Kobashi KC, Govier FE (2003) Perioperative complications: the first 140 polypropylene pubovaginal slings. *J Urol* **170:** 1918–21

Lane FE (1962) Repair of post-hysterectomy vaginal vault prolapse. *Obstet Gynecol* **20:** 72–7

Leron E, Stanton SL (2001) Sacrohysteropexy with synthetic mesh for the management of uterovaginal prolapse. *Brit J Obstet Gynaecol* **108:** 629–33.

Liu CY, Paek W (1993) Laparoscopic retropubic colposuspension (Burch procedure). *J Am Assoc Gynecol Laparosc* **1(1):** 31–5

Mahendran D, Prashar S *et al* (1996) Laparoscopic sacrocolpopexy in the management of vaginal vault prolapse. *Gynaecol Endosc* **5:** 217–22

Maher CF, Carey MP *et al* (2001) Laparoscopic suture hysteropexy for uterine prolapse. *Obstet Gynecol* **97:** 1010–4

Mallipeddi PK, Steele AC *et al* (2001) Anatomic and functional outcome of vaginal paravaginal repair in the correction of anterior vaginal wall prolapse. *Int Urogynecol J Pelvic Floor Dysfunct* **12(2):** 83–8

Marshall V, Marchetti A *et al* (1949) The correction of stress incontinence by simple vesicurethral suspension. *Surg Gynecol Obstet* **88:** 509

McLennan MT (2004) Transurethral resection of transvaginal tape. *Int Urogynecol J Pelvic Floor Dysfunct* **15:** 360–2

Mellier G, Benayed B *et al* (2004) Suburethral tape via the obturator route: is the TOT a simplification of the TVT? *Int Urogynecol J Pelvic Floor Dysfunct* **15:** 227–32

Miklos J, Kohli N (2000) Laparoscopic paravaginal repair plus Burch colposuspension: review and descriptive technique. *Urology* **56:** 64–69

Moehrer B, Ellis G *et al* (2002) Laparoscopic colposuspension for urinary incontinence in women. *Cochrane Database Syst Rev* **1:** CD002239

Morley G, DeLancey J (1988) Sacrospinous ligament fixation for eversion of the vagina. *Am J Obstet Gynecol* **158:** 872–81

Nezhat CH, Nezhat F *et al* (1994) Laparoscopic sacral colpopexy for vaginal vault prolapse. *Obstet Gynecol* **84:** 885–8

Nichols D (1982) Sacrospinous fixation for massive eversion of the vagina. *Am J Obstet Gynecol* **142:** 901–4

Nieminem K, Heinonen P (2001) Sacrospinous ligament fixation for massive genital prolapse in women aged over 80 years. *Brit J Obstet Gynecol* **108:** 817–21

Olsen AL, Smith VJ *et al* (1997) Epidemiology of surgically managed pelvic organ prolapse and urinary incontinence. *Obstet Gynecol* **89:** 501–6

Ou C, Presthus J *et al* (1993) Laparoscopic bladder neck suspension using hernia mesh and surgical staples. *J Laparoendosc Surg* **3:** 563–6

Palma P, Dambros M *et al* (2005) The Ibero-American experience with a re-adjustable minimally invasive sling. *B J Urol* **95:** 341–

Persson J, Wolner-Hanssen P (2000) Laparoscopic Burch colposuspension for stress urinary incontinence: a randomised comparison of one or two sutures on each side of the urethra. *Obstet Gynecol* **95:** 151–5

Petros P, Ulmsten U (1990) An integral theory of female urinary incontinence. Experimental and clinical considerations. *Acta Obstet Gynecol Scand* **69(Suppl):** 153

Petros P (200) Vault prolapse: Restoration of dynamic vaginal supports by infracoccygeal sacropexy, an axial day-case vaginal procedure. *Internat Urogynaecol J* **12:** 296–303

Pickard R, Reaper J *et al* (2003) Periurethral injection therapy for urinary incontinence in women. *Cochrane Database Syst Rev* **2:** CD003881.

Ross J, Galen D *et al* (2002) A prospective multisite study of radiofrequency bipolar energy for treatment of genuine stress incontinence. *J Amer Assoc Gynecol Laparosc* **9:** 493–9

Speights S, Moore R *et al* (2000) Frequency of lower urinary tract injury at laparoscopic Burch and paravaginal repair. *J Am Assoc Gynecol Laparosc* **7:** 515–8

Stevenson K, Cholhan H *et al* (1999) Lower urinary tract injury during the Burch procedure. Is there a role for routine cystoscopy? *Am J Obstet Gynecol* **181:** 35–8

Su TH, Wang KG *et al* (1997) Prospective comparison of laparoscopic and traditional colposuspension in the treatment of genuine stress incontinence. *Acta Obstet Gynecol* **76:** 576–82

Sze EHM, Karram MM (1997) Transvaginal repair of vault prolapse: a review. *Obstetr Gynecol* **89:** 466–75

Tanagho EA (1976) Colpocystourethropexy: The way we do it. *J Urol* **116:** 751

Tsivian A, Mogutin B *et al* (2004) Tension-free vaginal tape procedure for the treatment of female stress urinary incontinence: long-term results. *J Urol* **172:** 998–1000

Ulmsten U, Henriksson L *et al* (1996) Ambulatory surgical procedure under local anaesthetic for the treatment of female urinary incontinence. *Int Urogynecol J* **7:** 81–6

Ulmsten U, Henriksson L *et al* (2001) The basic understanding and clinical results of tension-free vaginal tape for stress urinary incontinence. *Urologe A* **40:** 269–73

Üstün Y, Engin-Üstün Y *et al* (2003) Tension-free vaginal tape compared with Burch urethropexy. *J Am Assoc Gynecol Laparosc* **10:** 386–9

Valpas A, Kivela A *et al* (2004) Tension-free vaginal tape and laparoscopic mesh colposuspension for stress urinary incontinence. *Obstet Gynecol* **104:** 42–9

Vancaile T, Schussler W (1991) Laparoscopic bladder-neck suspension. *J Laparoendosc Surg* **1:** 169–73

Visco AG, Weidner AC *et al* (2001) Vaginal mesh erosion after abdominal sacral colpopexy. *Am J Obstet and Gynaecol* **184:** 297–302

Wai CY, Atnip SD *et al* (2004) Urethral erosion of tension-free vaginal tape presenting as recurrent stress urinary incontinence. *Int Urogynecol J Pelvic Floor Dysfunct* **15:** 353–5

Ward KL, Hilton P (2004) UK and Ireland TVT Trial Group A prospective multicenter randomized trial of tension-free vaginal tape and colposuspension for primary urodynamic stress incontinence: two-year follow-up. *Am J Obstet Gynecol* **190:** 324–31

Washington J, Somers K (2003) Laparoscopic paravaginal repair: a new technique using mesh and staples. *Journal of the Society of Laparoendoscopic Surgeons* **7:** 301–3

Weidner AC, Cundiff GW *et al* (1997) Sacral osteomyelitis: an unusual complication of abdominal sacral colpopexy. *Obstet Gynecol* **90:** 689–91

Young S, Daman J *et al* (2001) Vaginal paravaginal repair: one year outcomes. *Am J Obstet Gynecol* **185:** 1360–7

Zullo F, Palomba S *et al* (2001) Laparoscopic Burch colposuspension: a randomised controlled trial comparing two transperitoneal surgical techniques. *Obstet Gynecol* **98:** 783–8

CHAPTER 12

Robotics in surgery

A Darzi, PS Sains, A Zivanovic

Robots in surgery can be classified into various groups according to the tasks they carry out. Currently available robotic systems range from powered robots which act as passive tool holders, active robots which carry out complex motions and interact with the patient, synergistic robotic systems that allow the surgeon to have 'hands on' and feel the operative forces applied by the instruments, telemanipulator robots which downscale movements with accuracy and remote-controlled telemedicine robots that allow experts to be virtually present at the patient's bedside. The distinction between computer aided surgery and classification of surgical robots is discussed and examples of each type of robot are given.

Introduction

Research into surgical robotics began approximately twenty years ago with the use of a standard industrial robot in a neurosurgical procedure, (Kwoh *et al*, 1988) but it is only over the last ten years that they have begun to be used regularly in operating rooms. This chapter will give an overview of various ways robots are used in surgery, with examples of particular systems. First, we should define what we mean by the term 'surgical robot'. This seemingly simple task is fraught with difficulty as it hard enough to reach consensus about the meaning of the word 'robot'. Perhaps Engelberger (McKerrow, 1991) put it best when he said 'You know one when you see one'. However, this is not sufficiently precise for our purpose, so it is perhaps best to accept the suggestion put forward by Prof. Brian Davies (Davies, 2000) of Imperial College London: 'A surgical robot is a powered, computer-controlled manipulator, with artificial sensing, that can be reprogrammed to move and position tools to carry out a range of surgical tasks'.

The motivation behind the use of robots in surgery is to improve the outcome of medical procedures by combining the advantages of robots (eg. high precision positioning of tools, repeatability) with the best qualities of a human surgeon (eg. intelligence, responding to change). Thus, surgical robots are rarely intended to replace the surgeon, but rather to work as an intelligent tool to assist him/her in carrying out an operation. In order to achieve this goal, robotic systems generally require preoperative imaging, computer modeling and registration of the robotic instruments and patient anatomy to the imaging so that the robot 'knows' where the patient is in 3-D space.

A Darzi, PS Sains, A Zivanovic

Computer assisted surgery

A distinction should be made between robot assisted surgery and computer assisted surgery (CAS). CAS relies upon the surgeon manually positioning the instruments, whereas in robotic surgery the tools are positioned by a motorized system. CAS systems are mainly used to track instruments or anatomy by optical or magnetic methods, or by monitoring the joint positions of a passive manipulator. The resulting three dimensional coordinates enable the tool to be represented on a computer screen in relation to the operative anatomy. The anatomy must, before this, undergo imaging. This is commonly either computer tomography (CT), ultrasound (US) or magnetic resonance imaging (MRI) and the resulting images are used to construct a three dimensional model of the target anatomy. Fixed recognizable regions of the anatomy are then 'registered' to the model by the tracking system. This approach is most suited to orthopedic surgery as bone can be clamped and fixed. It is then assumed that the target anatomy is fixed during the operative procedure. With tissues that undergo constant movement during a procedure the concept of 'dynamic referencing' is applied where the constant tracking and adjustment of the display occurs as reference points change.

Robotic systems

Surgical robots can be classified as:
- Passive tool holders or manipulators
- Active robots
- Synergistic systems
- Telemanipulator systems
- Telemedicine robotic systems

Passive tool holder robots (powered)

One of the earliest applications of surgical powered robots was use in holding fixtures in static situations, allowing the surgeon to locate instrumentation though them. An example of this was the use of an industrial robot in neurosurgery (Kwoh *et al*, 1988). A stereotactic frame attached to the patient's head was registered by the robot to the patient as well as the robot to the preoperative CT scan. The robot then moved to the desired position and locked into position allowing safe and accurate drilling of the skull. A biopsy of the brain tumor was then carried out. The surgeon's movements were restricted to linear insertions of the instruments through the fixed robot.

Active robots

Active robots allow powered interaction with the patient and can allow more complex motions than the powered robots used as passive tool holders.

Laparoscopic camera holders

Traditionally the surgeon has the use of an assistant to hold and move the laparoscopic camera. The assistant attempts to predict the surgeon's movements and anticipate the view that is required. Not only can this be a difficult task but the view provided may not be ideal because of tremor and positioning of the horizon. The AESOP (Automated Endoscopic System for Optimal Positioning) (Mittelstadt *et al*, 1993) robotic arm is shown below.

The demands on the robot to hold and move the camera are extensive as movements encompassing pitch, roll, yaw, advance and withdraw have to be made. These movements are made about a fulcrum at the entry site into the body cavity. Control of the camera is achieved by foot pedals, head sensors or more recently voice activation.

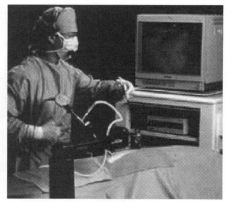

Figure 12.1: The AESOP camera holder robotic arm (Automated Endoscopic System for Optimal Positioning).

Orthopedic hip surgery

There are commercially available orthopedic robots (eg. 'Robodoc', Integrated Surgical Supplies Ltd, Sacramento, USA) (Sackier and Wang, 1994) which carry a high speed rotary cutter at the tip. Furthermore, the robot has force sensors at the wrist. This allows reaming of the femoral bone cavity in preparation for the stem of the hip prosthesis to be implanted.

Preoperatively, a computer model of the proposed implant is superimposed over a three dimensional model of the hip. This allows satisfactory positioning of the implant on the three dimensional model prior to any incision being made. The patient's leg. is then held by means of clamps, in that way fixing the femur. The predetermined movements, as planned on the three dimensional model, of the robot are then executed. The movements of the robot within the femur can also be displayed on the computer simultaneously.

Urology-prostate surgery

Transurethral resection of the prostate (TURP) is a common procedure which is carried out for benign enlargement of the prostate, resulting in urinary outflow obstruction. The conventional surgical treatment is performed via the urethra through an endoscope. The prostate, which is held in a fixed position by the pelvis, is then de-bulked by the use of a cauterized loop.

The 'Probot' (Ng *et al*, 1993) robot (Mechatronics in Medicine Group, Imperial College London) is an active robotic system for prostatectomies. The robot is equipped with an ultrasound probe that allows direct evaluation of the prostate size. The images produced by the ultrasound can be evaluated by the surgeon and the tissue that requires resection can be targeted. The ultrasound probe is then removed and the robot is fitted with a cutter. The ultrasound images are used to construct a three dimensional model and the cutting trajectories of the robot are defined. Debulking of the prostate can then be carried out.

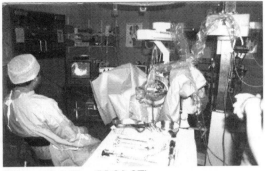

Figure 12.2: The 'PROBOT'

Synergistic systems

Synergistic systems allow the surgeon to hold a force-controlled handle located on the robot, which also carries a tool. The user imparts a force on the handle and the robot is powered to move in the specified direction. If the tool approaches a volume of space previously defined to be forbidden, the robot prevents the further motion in that direction. This concept is called 'active constraints'. The synergistic system allows the surgeon's skills and judgment to be combined with the constraints provided by the robot, allowing an accurate and safe operation.

The 'Acrobot' orthopedic robot

The Acrobot (Davies *et al*, 1997) is a robot developed for knee replacement surgery at Imperial College London and is now being developed by a spin-out company of the same name. CT scans of the patient's leg. are taken preoperatively and a 3D computer model is constructed on screen. The surgeon chooses a suitable prosthesis and overlays it on the computer model. The system calculates the constraints (eg. the cutting planes). During the operation, the patient's knee is fixed in position. The position of the knee is registered to the robot's coordinate system. The surgeon is then able to control the cutter by hand within the constrained area, providing accurate shaping for the prosthesis to fit into. Furthermore, as the surgeon can feel the forces experienced by the robot cutting instrument he is able to judge the speed and force that need to be applied. This avoids damage to vulnerable areas such as soft bone.

Telemanipulator systems

Telemanipulator systems can also be described as 'master-slave' systems. The master is separated from the slave and consists of a control, for example, a joystick. The slave mimics the movements that are carried out at the master system by the surgeon. Although, at present, the master system is generally placed in proximity to the slave, it is possible to operate it from a remote location, over dedicated communication channels.

Telemanipulator systems allow the larger movements of the surgeon at the master to be scaled down to micro movements with smaller forces of the slave instruments.

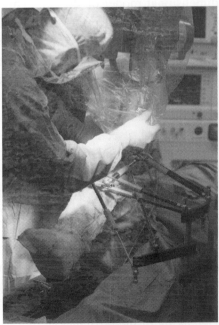

Figure 12.3: The 'ACROBOT'

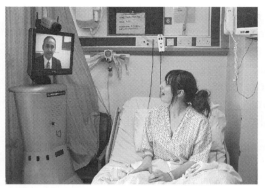

Figure 12.4: Expert availability via a remote robotic system

The da Vinci (Intuitive Surgical, USA) and ZEUS (Computer Motion, USA) systems.

The da Vinci (Carpentier *et al*, 1999) and ZEUS *(www.fda.gov/fdac/features/2002/302_bots.html (accessed 2005)* incorporate the use of a robotic arm holding an endoscope with two other arms carrying the surgical tools. The tools have been designed to give a 'wristing motion' allowing greater degrees of freedom within the body cavity. At present, neither system allows the surgeon to 'feel' the tissue. This is termed 'haptics' and is currently at the forefront of research into force-sensing systems at the slave which are then fed back to the master and hence the surgeon.

Telemedicine robotic systems

Telemedicine has been described as the 'the use of electronic signals to transfer medical data (photographs, x-ray images, audio, patient records, videoconferences, etc.) from one site to another, via the Internet, intranets, personal computers (PCs), satellites, or videoconferencing telephone equipment, in order to improve access to healthcare.'

Telemedicine systems have traditionally consisted of 'static' hardware consisting of a camera and personal computer or television screen. Due to the static nature of the systems, the patient needs to be brought to the camera rather than the clinician being able to visit the patient or patients on a ward setting.

The advent of remotely controlled robots which can be controlled by the clinician allows the teleconsultation to be patient-centered. The clinician is able to review the patient by visiting him/her remotely.

Remote presence technology (InTouch Health, USA)

The RP6 robot is a remotely controlled robot that has a camera and screen mounted on it. The robot is battery powered and relies upon wireless technology and broadband internet connections for its control. The clinician is able to log into a desktop control station consisting of a dual monitor screen, computer, camera, speakers and a control joystick. The monitor at the control station displays the view of the camera on the robot and the screen on the robot displays the view of the camera mounted at the control station and directed at the user's face and thereby allows real-time audiovisual communication. The user is able to move the robot mounted camera and use zoom facilities to provide the required views of the patient or observations.

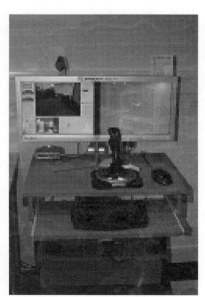

Figure 12.5: The remote robot control station

The main control joystick enables the clinician to move the robot in multidirectional manner. This is achieved by three motorized runners which move the robot. Collision of the robot with objects is minimized by the use of sensors located at ankle and knee height on the robot. The sensors display proximity of the robot to objects on the control panel screen. When very close to an object, the sensors disable the motors thereby avoiding collision.

The ability of a clinician to be virtually present may carry significant advantages in patient care and medical education by increasing the availability of senior personnel.

Key points for *Chapter 12*

- A distinction should be made between robot assisted surgery and computer assisted surgery (CAS). CAS relies upon the surgeon manually positioning the instruments, whereas in robotic surgery the tools are positioned by a motorized system.

- Robots have the potential to be autonomous and carry out repetitive actions without fatigue and move in complex pathways with accuracy.

- Robotic systems can be classified into passive tool holders or manipulators, active robots, synergistic systems, telemanipulator systems and telemedicine robotic systems.

- Passive robots act as a guiding fixture for the operating surgeon because they can be safely locked into position.

- Active robots perform autonomous actions which are supervised by the surgeon.

- Synergistic systems allow the surgeon to hold a force-controlled handle located on the robot, which also carries a tool. This allows the surgeon to feel the forces exerted on the target tissue.

- Telemanipulator systems are based on a 'master-slave' concept where the surgeon's hand movements are downscaled to accurate, tremor free micro movements at the slave instrument tip.

- Telemedicine robots allow remote availability of an expert at the patient's bedside by means of internet and wireless technologies.

- Further collaboration between medical personnel, engineers, computer scientists will allow for smaller more sophisticated robots.

References

Carpentier A, Loulmet D *et al* (1999) Computer assisted cardiac surgery. *Lancet* **353:** 379–80.

Davies B (2000). A review of robotics in surgery. *Proc Inst Mech Eng [H]* **214(1):** 129–40.

Davies BL, Lin WJ *et al* (1997) Active compliance in robotic surgery—the use of force control as a dynamic constraint. *Proc Inst Mech Eng, J Engineer Med* **211(H4):** 285–292

Kwoh YS, Hou J *et al* (1988) A robot with improved absolute positioning accuracy for CT guided stereotactic brain surgery. IEEE Trans Biomed. *Engineer* **35(2):** 153–61

McKerrow PJ (1991) *Introduction to robotics.* Addison-Wesley New York

Mittelstadt BD, Kazanzides P, *et al* (1993) Robotic surgery: achieving predictable results in an unpredictable environment. In: Proceedings of 6th International Conference on Advanced Robotics Tokyo: 367–372.

Ng WS, Davies BL *et al* (1993) A firsthand experience in transurethral resection of prostate. IEEE, EMBS J: 120–125

Sackier JM, Wang Y (1994). Robotically assisted laparoscopic surgery: from concept to development. *Surg Endosc* **8:** 63–66

www.fda.gov/fdac/features/2002/302_bots.html (accessed 2005)

CHAPTER 13

Robotic versus pure laparoscopic surgery

JV Joseph, R Madeb, HRH Patel

Robotic surgery has sent an exciting wave through the world of medicine It has transcended from the big screen to local hospitals where it has significantly improved patient outcomes. The constant improvement in robotic technology has allowed surgeons to perform complex tasks, not previously possible with robots. The improved optics and engineering provided by the newer robotic systems has increased the application of robots in a number of disciplines, bringing minimally invasive surgery within the reach of surgeons without prior laparoscopic or robotic experience.

With continued technological improvement, the advantages of the robot will be amplified as the manufacturers overcome the limitations. In a number of surgical disciplines, robots are poised to redefine the gold standard, and not just be a fleeting phenomenon.

Introduction

No other emerging technological tool has taken the surgical arena by storm, as robotic surgery has. Despite the current lack of practical applications in all surgical subspecialties and its costly operating system, robotic surgery has largely been patient driven secondary to intense marketing. It still remains to be determined whether robotic surgery can leap from surgical ability to surgical practicality. Currently, the three major fields of surgery that have embraced robotic systems are general, cardiac, and urologic surgery (*Table 13.1*). Its advancement in surgical subspecialties such as cardiac and urologic surgery stems from the limitations general laparoscopy has in these fields. To date, there is no procedure in the urologic and cardiac subspecialties that equates to the relative ease of laparoscopic cholecystectomy. Laparoscopic skills in urologic and cardiac surgery have been slow to evolve and are mainly developed in highly specialized academic institutions. Robotic surgery has greatly reduced the technical challenge and learning curve needed to perform minimally invasive surgery and extends the potential for a conventional 'open surgeon' to develop these skills.

Table 13.1: Current surgical applications of robotic surgery by speciality

Urology	Cardiac	General Surgery	Other
Prostatectomy	Mitral valve repair	Cholecystectomy	Tubal ligation
Pyeloplasty	CABG	Nissen fundoplication	Tubal re-anastomosis
Nephrectomy	Mammary artery harvest	Heller myotomy	Ovarian resection
Adrenalectomy		Gastric bypass	Spinal surgery
Cystectomy		Splenectomy	

Advantages of robot assisted surgery compared to conventional laparoscopy

Laparoscopic surgery has afforded all subspecialties of surgery the possibility of performing major surgery with a minimally invasive approach. Initial benefits from laparoscopic surgery seen with earlier case series included a shorter convalescence, decreased postoperative pain, increased cosmesis, and earlier resumption of oral intake and daily activities. Certain procedures such as laparoscopic cholecystectomy, tubal ligation, and nephrectomy have become gold standard in many institutions and are the primary choice for surgical options.

Despite the wide acceptance of laparoscopy by many surgical subspecialties, technical limitations exist. Laparoscopic surgery in general is hampered by a limited range of motion, 2-D visualization, impaired hand-eye coordination, and reduced tactile motion. The reduction in range of motion exists because laparoscopic surgery is based on a fixed port system. The fixed trocar position determines the angle at which the instrument may move. Thus, the only motion possible with an instrument at a fixed port in the abdominal wall is rotation, pitch, yaw, and insertion. This is commonly referred as having 4-degrees of freedom. Another major obstacle is inability to have 3-D vision with laparoscopic surgery. The monocular camera coupled with the absence of shadows make it almost impossible for spatial and depth perception. This contributes to the surgeon's improper hand-eye coordination, dexterity and misalignment. This is crucial with small, tedious anastomotic surgical maneuvers, such as urethrovesical anastomosis, pyeloplasty and microsurgical techniques.

Although different maneuvers have been described by skilled laparoscopic specialists to overcome these problems, these limitations have not allowed conventional trained surgeons to embrace laparoscopy. The advancement of robotic systems, such as the daVinci robot, has addressed these problems and has overcome most of these obstacles. In fact, case series of open conventional surgeons transformed to laparoscopic minimally invasive surgeons have been reported in the urologic literature. In our center, we use the daVinci surgical system, as do most of the current centers actively embracing surgical robots. The advantages afforded by the da Vinci robot include increased dexterity, restoration of hand–eye coordination, ergonomic positioning, 3-D visualization and motion scaling. These benefits have not only made difficult laparoscopic procedures easier, they have allowed technically unfeasible procedures with laparoscopic approach feasible.

The robotic system enhances dexterity and hand-eye coordination in several ways. The highly specialized instruments with increased degree of freedom exhibited by the 'mechanical wrist' of the robotic unit allow the surgeon to hold and manipulate the tissues in different planes. Furthermore, the robot filters hand tremor and can perform motion scaling. Motion scaling refers to motion relationship between the master–slave system causing large movements at the control grips to be transformed into micro movements inside the patient. If a motion scale is set 5:1, the motion will move the tool 1mm inside the abdomen for every 5mm of motion at the master console. This allows for fine precision needed with tedious and fine maneuvers. Possibly, the biggest enhancement of dexterity and hand–eye coordination comes from the 3-D imaging system. The robotic unit is armed with a high-resolution three-dimensional endoscope consisting of two three-chip charged-coupled cameras with two high-intensity illuminators ensuring a bright 3-D image of the operative field. The computer image can generate a 5 to 10 times magnification according to the distance of the endoscope from the object in the operative field. Overall, the 3-D view with depth perception is a marked improvement from conventional laparoscopy. Moreover, the ability for the surgeon to control the focus and zoom from the surgeon's console eliminates the need for an additional person to control the camera as in conventional laparoscopy. These benefits offered by the surgical robot all contribute increased dexterity and a much improved operative experience for both surgeon and patient.

Disadvantages of robotic surgery

Although, the robotic experience is safe, feasible, invigorating and reminiscent of surgical experiences from a science fiction novel, it is not without disadvantages. The most apparent is the price of one million US dollars. Besides the initial cost of investment, maintenance costs can add up to nearly one quarter of a million dollars yearly. The instruments used with the daVinci are reusable, but have a set number of uses preset by the manufacturer. Once the maximum number of uses is reached, the instrument is automatically disabled, and must be replaced. These costs limit the widespread adoption of the daVinci robot at many centers.

Another disadvantage of this system is the size of the machine and the technical assistance needed to set-up the machine. The daVinci robot's size matches its heavy price and requires significant space in today's already overcrowded operating room. Moreover, the system requires trained personnel with the robot's set-up; and set-up times of over one hour in the initial stages have been reported. At our center however, we have had set-up times in the 10–15 minute range with increasing experience. Whether miniaturization or the use of wall-mountable robots will help decrease set-up times, remain a question.

Only time will determine the fate of the future surgical robot. Another disadvantage with the current surgical system is the lack of compatible surgical instruments and equipment. This too is a transient disadvantage and will be resolved with newer technological advancements. Most of the

Table 13.2: Comparison of conventional laparoscopic *versus* robotic surgery

Type of Surgery	Advantages	Disadvantages
Laparoscopic	■ Well-developed ■ Proven efficacy with sufficient long-term data reported ■ Becoming more affordable and readily available in multiple small and large centers	■ No 3-D visualization ■ No tactile sensation ■ Limited range of motion (4-degrees of freedom)
Robotic	■ 3-D visualization ■ Improved dexterity ■ Increased range of motion (7-degrees of freedom) ■ Elimination of physiologic tremor ■ Ability for scale motion ■ Ergonomic and untiring ■ Possibility for tele-surgery ■ Possibility for microsurgery and microanastomosis	■ Very expensive with high set-up and maintenance cost ■ Newer technology with unproven cost-benefit ■ High set-up cost with the need for additional trained staff ■ Large size of the robot ■ Highly specialized instruments ■ No tactile sensation

disadvantages identified will be remedied with time and improvements in technology. In addition, long-term feasibility, oncological and cost-benefit studies are needed to fix the role of robotic surgical systems in the surgical arena. *Table 13.2* compares the advantages and disadvantages between conventional laparoscopic and robotic surgery.

Clinical application of robotic surgery

Although the daVinci robot was first introduced in cardiac surgery, it has found its main application in urologic pelvic surgeries. Radical prostatectomy is by far the most common procedure performed using the daVinci robot. At a number of institutions, it is used exclusively for urologic procedures.

The evolution of radical prostatectomy from open conventional radical surgery to laparoscopy and finally robotic surgery is an excellent procedure to show the rapid inclusion of robotic surgery. Radical bilateral nerve sparing retropubic prostatectomy described and modified by Patrick Walsh is the most commonly performed operation for localized prostate cancer (Walsh, 1998). This procedure was performed only via an open approach until 1992 when Shuessler reported the first laparoscopic radical prostatectomy. Due to the difficulties encountered, the procedure was abandoned (Schuesssler *et al*, 1992; Schuessler *et al*, 1997). In the late 1990's, however there was renewed interest in laparoscopic radical prostatectomy after Guillonneau and Vallancien reported their success performing this procedure with clinical efficacy, and efficiency comparable to the standard open approach (Guillonneau *et al*, 1999). The combination of less postoperative morbidity, improved cosmesis, shorter convalescence and comparable oncological outcome has increased interest in minimally invasive surgery, and lured many patients away from the conventional retropubic prostatectomy. Comparative studies of laparoscopic versus open retropubic prostatectomy have been performed which reveal comparative oncological results with decreased morbidity and shorter convalescence (Guillonneau and Vallancien, 2000).

Since the reports by Guillonneau *et al*, various centers worldwide regularly perform laparoscopic prostatectomy as a first line surgical treatment for clinically localized prostate cancer. Multiple studies from both highly academic to private institutions have shown feasibility and satisfactory early functional and oncological results (Guillonneau and Vallancien, 2000; Dahl *et al*, 2002). Despite its feasibility, the procedure has been described as lengthy and technically challenging with a steep learning curve. Problems with conventional laparoscopy including 2-D vision, inadequate dexterity, maneuverability, and ergonomics hindered laparoscopic prostatectomy from becoming the new gold standard.

During the last five years advances in laparoscopic equipment and technique, most notably, the addition of the daVinci (Intuitive Surgical, Mountain View, California) surgical system have resulted in significant progress in the development of minimally invasive surgery for localized prostate cancer. The barriers of conventional laparoscopy have been overcome, with several institutions reporting successful outcomes in large series of patients (Menon *et al*, 2002). The vesicourethral anastomosis which requires advanced laparoscopic skills that only few urologists possess, had become a quick and easy step. The anastomosis performed at the end of the procedure, when the surgeon is tired after standing for several hours, can be performed with the surgeon, sitting, with his head and hands resting comfortably on the console.

The robotic prostatectomy procedure relies on the same principles of the anatomic radical prostatectomy as described by Patrick Walsh (Menon *et al*, 2002). However, it could now be approached in a timely, efficient, and minimally invasive manner. The advantages of robotic surgery, including ergonomics, 3-D visualization, and ability to perform intracorporeal suturing has led to reproducibility and excellent early results.

At the University Of Rochester Medical Center, we routinely performed a total extraperitoneal approach to the removal of the prostate, using the daVinci robot. Initially, we used a pure laparoscopic approach based on the Institute Mutualiste Montsouris experience, described elsewhere in this book. After multiple modifications, we developed a total extraperitoneal approach and found this procedure to be technically feasible and reproducible. In 2003, we extrapolated our procedure to incorporate the daVinci robotic surgical system (Joseph *et al*, 2005).

Current operative outcomes

We have performed over 500 extraperitoneal robotic radical prostatectomies with a zero open conversion rate. Our patients experience a high continence rate with 93% of them being fully continent (no pads) by three months, and 29% of them having immediate (upon catheter removal at one week post-op) control of continence. Of patients who had bilateral nerve-sparing, 28/45 (62.2%) had mild or no Erectile Dysfunction (ED) within six to eight months post-surgery and all expressed satisfaction with their current sexual function or rate of improvement after robotic prostatectomy.

Robot-assisted extraperitoneal prostatectomy has become our preferred surgical approach. The precision and improved visualization of the robot compliments the surgeon's skills, while the abdominal cavity and potential associated morbidity are avoided. Overall, the robot-assisted extraperitoneal approach offers equivalent oncological and functional results along with decreased transfusion rates and shorter convalescence compared to the open conventional technique. They are generally discharged home in less than twenty-four hours, with catheter removal one week after surgery. The advantages of the robot have contributed to its increased use at a number of medical centers.

Conclusion

Laparoscopic surgery has revolutionized the surgical arena. The benefits of robotic surgery such as increased dexterity, 3-D visualization and improved hand–eye coordination has allowed new approaches in extirpative and reconstructive urologic surgery. Moreover, in today's competitive healthcare market many organizations are seeking 'the cutting-edge experience' and are investing in this technology. Robotic surgery will continue to be sought after and will remain a very attractive option. However, it should be noted that although attractive, robotic surgery is still in its infancy. Surgeons interested in robotic surgery should receive proper training to ensure the best outcomes for their patients. The limitations of the daVinci robot will be resolved as time goes by, and newer technology is brought forth. Ultimately, randomized studies including feasibility, outcomes and cost–benefit analysis will come forth to help determine its place in our surgical armamentarium, beyond the marketing phenomenon. Comparing pure laparoscopic surgery with daVinci robotic surgery, the former is most likely a transitional technique between open surgery and robot assisted surgery.

Key points for *Chapter 13*

- Robots help surgeons overcome the limitations of traditional laparoscopy.
- The da Vinci robot is the most popular unit in use.
- Advantages of the daVinci robot include increased dexterity, hand-eye coordination, ergonomic positioning, 3-dimensional visualization, and motion scaling.
- Robotic surgeons rely on visual cues, due to the absence of proprioception, or haptic feedback.
- The high initial and maintenance costs of the robot limits its application to only large medical centers.
- The shortcomings of current robotic units will be eliminated with continued improvement of surgical technology.
- Radical prostatectomy has been an excellent application of the daVinci robot.
- Proper laparoscopic training is necessary prior to starting robotic assisted surgery.

References

Dahl DM, L'esperance JO *et al* (2002) Laparoscopic radical prostatectomy: Initial 70 cases at a US university medical center. *Urology* **60:** 859

Guillonneau B, Cathelineau X *et al* (1999) Laparoscopic radical prostatectomy:technical and early oncological assessment of 40 operations. *Eur Urol* **36:** 14–20

Guillonneau B, Vallancien GV (2000) Laparoscopic radical prostatectomy: the Montsouris technique. *J Urol* **163:** 1643–9

Joseph J, Madeb RM *et al* (2005) Laparoscopic radical prostatectomy *vs.* robotic assisted radical prostatectomy: what are the differences. *BJU Int* **96(1):** 39–42

Joseph JV, Madeb R *et al* (2005) Laparoscopic Radical Prostatectomy following Laparoscopic Bilateral Mesh Hernia Repair. *J Soc Laparoendo Surg* **9(3):** 368–9

Joseph JV, Patel HRH (2004) Transperitoneal or Extraperitoneal Approach for Laparoscopic Radical Prostatectomy: A False Debate Over a Real Challenge (letter). *J Urol* **172**

Marescaux J, Smith MK *et al* (2001) Telerobotic laparoscopic cholecystectomy: initial clinical experience with 25 patients. *Ann Surg* **234:** 1–7

Menon M, Tewari A *et al* (2002) Prospective comparison of radical retropubic prostatectomy and robot assisted anatomic prostatectomy: the Vattikuti Urology Institute experience. *Urology* **60:** 864–8

Patel HRH, Madeb R *et al* (2004) Extraperitoneal robotic prostatectomy: the Rochester method. *BJU Int* **94(S2):** 160 (abstract V-5.02) 11

Paul HA, Bargar WL *et al* (1992) Development of a surgical robot for cementless total hip arthroplasty. *Clin Orthop* **285:** 57–66

Schuessler WW, Kavoussi LR *et al* (1992) Laparoscopic radical prostatectomy:initial case report. *J Urol* **147:** 246A

Schuessler WW, Schulam PG *et al* (1997) Laparoscopic radical prostatectomy: initial short-term experience. *Urology* **50:** 854–7

Walsh PC (1998) Anatomic radical prostatectomy:evolution of the surgical technique. *J Urol* **160:** 2418–24

CHAPTER 14

Biomedical microrobotics: the future of minimally invasive treatments

KB Yesin, BJ Nelson

The emerging field of biomedical microrobotics can be described as the development of highly integrated mechatronic systems that are positioned inside the body for minimally invasive medical diagnosis and intervention. It combines the established theory and techniques of robotics with the exciting new tools enabled by Micro-Electro-Mechanical-Systems (MEMS) technology to significantly improve the quality of our lives. This chapter presents a short overview of this field, summarizing different application areas, and related challenges. The first commercial applications were capsule endoscopy systems; pill sized robots for the inspection of the gastrointestinal path. Recent international projects are targeting cardiovascular, ophthalmic and urologic applications. These sub-millimetre sized robots require the highest possible level of integration through modular, hybrid MEMS designs. Storage of energy is another challenge at this scale. We analyze the possibility of using externally generated magnetic fields for steering and actuation of these robots.

Introduction

'Microscopic sized robots, remote controlled inside the human body for medical diagnosis and intervention'. This could be the topic of a Hollywood blockbuster. It is no surprise that it was Hollywood to first 'realize' the idea of in-vivo micromachines in motion pictures such as *Fantastic Voyage* (1966) or *Inner Space* (1987). Since then, microsystems technology developed with ever increasing speed. Today, not only scenarists but also engineers are working to make it happen.

Micro-Electro-Mechanical-Systems (MEMS) is now a commercial technology with various sub-fields and a large variety of application areas. The acceleration sensor that triggers your car's airbag or the microscopic flipping mirrors that create the images from a digital projector are two examples of everyday MEMS. Usually, it is a combination of low cost, low power consumption and small size that makes a MEMS-based design the better choice compared to conventional technology. But MEMS can also be an enabling technology, opening new frontiers to science (Sun *et al*, 2005).

It is easy to notice challenging design issues when envisioning a medical microrobot for in-vivo application. It must be small, reliable and biocompatible. It must carry all of the necessary

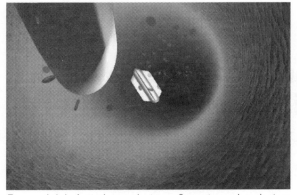

Figure 14.1: Artist's rendering of a microrobot being released into the bloodstream through a needle

tools and subsystems on-board. It must be removed from the target area of the patient's body in a 'non-invasive' manner.

The gastro-intestinal (GI) path took the early attention of researchers for being a suitable and important application area for such robots. This two-ended tunnel through the body which can tolerate relatively large sized objects was also where the first commercial systems were applied. (*www.rfnorika.com; www.givenimaging.com*) These untethered, endoscopic capsules are the size of a pill and are simply swallowed by the patient. They capture video images from the GI path with their imaging and illumination systems while naturally traveling through the path. Other researchers proposed robotic systems with locomotion and biopsy capabilities (Dario *et al*, 1996; Kim *et al*, 2003). Typically, robots built for the GI path are miniaturized mechatronic systems with many components of conventional design.

It is in the more challenging parts of the human body where truly microscopic sized robots would be needed that MEMS technology provides the only solution. Robots swimming in the blood stream or inside the vitreous humor (a clear, gel-like substance that fills the posterior cavity of the eye) have been envisioned (Mathieu *et al*, 2000; Yesin *et al*, 2004). A reoccurring theme with such microrobots is the use of ex-vivo generated magnetic fields to transfer energy to the robot. Whereas MEMS and VLSI technologies have accomplished the miniaturization of structural and electronic components, a corresponding breakthrough in energy storage was not achieved. This issue comes to the center-stage with sub-mm sized microrobots for cardiovascular or ophthalmic applications.

Magnetic actuation technology has been applied in biological systems for many years. A common application area is targeted drug delivery where magnetized carrier particles that are coated with various chemical agents are concentrated on specific target regions of the body using external magnetic fields (Hafeli *et al*, 1997; Holligan *et al*, 2003). A similar idea is used in magnetic cell separation where magnetized particles that are selectively attached to a targeted group of cells through their chemical composition are used to sort apart the cells (Zborowski *et al*, 1997). Individual magnetic beads of a few microns diameter have also been steered inside cells for the study of their mechanical properties (Amblard *et al*, 2000; Vicci, 2001) as well as for the manipulation of individual DNA molecules (Haber and Wirtz, 2000). These applications differ from drug targeting or cell separation in that

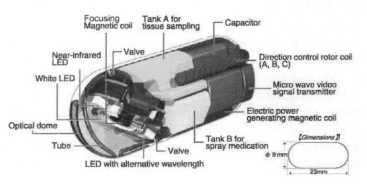

Figure 14.2: Capsule endoscope system from RFNorika www.rfnorika.com

precise and dynamic control of magnetic field vectors through real-time feedback is desired. Another area with similar requirements on field control is magnetically assisted stereotaxis to guide catherers inside the brain. (Grady *et al*, 1990; *www.stereotaxis.com*)

The basic equations describing magnetic interactions of matter give insight into the principle of magnetic steering and the consequences of miniaturization. The primary vectors that define the magnetostatic (ie. when the magnetic fields are DC or of low frequency) field in magnetized matter are the (external) magnetic field strength, H (A/m), the resulting magnetization of the matter $\mathbf{M}$ (A/m) and the net magnetic flux density $\mathbf{B}$ (Tesla). The relationship between these vectors is

$$\mathbf{B}=\mu_0(\mathbf{H+M})$$

where μ_0 is the magnetic permeability of free space defined as $4\pi \times 10^{-7}$ Tm/A. For the idealized case of linear, isotropic and homogeneous media the above relationship simplifies as

$$\mathbf{M}=\chi\mathbf{H}$$

$$\mathbf{B}=\mu_0(\mathbf{H}+\chi\mathbf{H})=\mu_0(1+\chi)\mathbf{H} = \mu_0 \mu_1 \mathbf{H}$$

where χ and μ_r are the susceptibility and relative permeability of the media, respectively. In general, these values are not constant but change with magnetization, putting a material dependent upper limit to the amount of magnetization known as the saturation magnetization $\mathbf{M_s}$. Within the saturation limits, the permeability can be thought as an amplification factor that creates a net magnetic field inside the matter through an external field.

The magnetic force and torque that are exerted on an object with uniform magnetization $\mathbf{M}$ in a magnetic field with flux density $\mathbf{B}$ are defined as

$$\mathbf{F}_m = V_m (\mathbf{M}.\Delta)\mathbf{B}$$

$$\mathbf{T}_m = V_m \mathbf{M} \times \mathbf{B}$$

where V_m is the volume of the magnetized object. Notice that the magnetic torque is dependent on $\mathbf{B}$ whereas the magnetic force is dependent on the gradient of $\mathbf{B}$. These equations also indicate that magnetic forces are volumetric. Therefore, the required field and field gradient to exert a certain torque and force on a magnetized object increases rapidly as the object gets smaller. In contrast, the viscous drag forces from the body fluids are related to the surface area of the robot, therefore, there is a disadvantage in terms of the necessary external magnetic field strengths as the robot's size goes smaller.

Another design challenge for a sub-mm sized microrobot is the high degree of integration that is needed. Most MEMS devices are designed to be components that are inserted into larger sized electro-mechanical systems. Even the system-on-a-chip type devices with integrated mechanical and electronic components need to be physically interfaced for power supply and data I/O. In contrast, the sub-mm sized medical microrobot must be micro-manufactured to its final form. The emerging technology of Hybrid MEMS, where individual MEMS components are combined through a robotic microassembly process, promises a solution (Yesin and Nelson, 2004). In a Hybrid MEMS design, different and incompatible manufacturing technologies

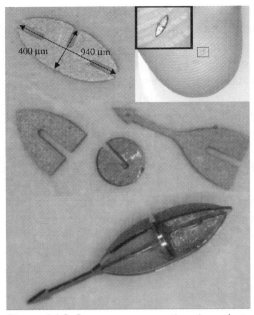

Figure 14.3: Prototype magnetic microrobot with Hybrid MEMS design.

(eg. Lithography, LIGA (Lithography Galvanoformung Abformung), Micro Opto Electro Mechanical Systems (MOEMS), Nanosystems) can be used together. By separately manufacturing the sub-components using the optimal technique and parameters, increased yields can be achieved. Most importantly, with three dimensional manipulation and assembly, the flat, 2.5-D shape limitations inherent in standard MEMS manufacturing methods can be overcome. With a 3-D geometry, more efficient use of allowed robot volume is possible.

A biomedical microrobot with a Hybrid MEMS design is being developed at the ETH Institute of Robotics and Intelligent Systems. The first area of application of this robot will be ophthalmic operations on the retina. *Figure 14.3* shows an early prototype microrobot with a three dimensional structure which was built to investigate hybrid MEMS assembly and magnetic steering concepts. The 50 μm thick nickel parts were manufactured using an electroplating process and bonded with UV activated glue. The 'winged-ellipsoid' shape of the robot has an axis of symmetry along the long axis of the ellipsoid. An external magnetic field acts to align and pull the robot along this axis (ie magnetic torque and force) due to the shape anisotropy effect, much like a needle always becoming magnetized along its long axis. On the other hand, the winged shape acts to reduce the sideways drift of the microrobot by increasing the fluid drag along the axes perpendicular to the long axis.

An important issue related to the control of a magnetic microrobot is the nonlinear nature of the field and field gradients that are created by electromagnet coils or by permanent magnets. The field from an air-core solenoid coil along its axis is roughly proportional to the inverse square of the distance to the solenoid. In this case the torque and force on the soft magnetic material are proportional to the fourth and fifth inverse power of the distance respectively. To appreciate the effect of this nonlinearity, one could try to levitate a small metallic object in a water-filled cup by moving a permanent magnet close and afar. It is not possible to stabilize such a system without high bandwidth feedback and actuation. One way of reducing these nonlinearities is to create uniform magnetic fields and field gradients using various coil

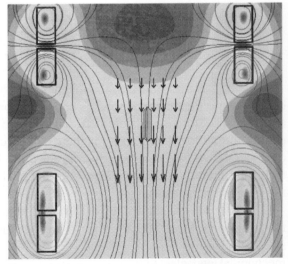

Figure 14.4: Superimposed magnetic field generated by concentric Maxwell and Helmholtz coils. This configuration enables independent control of magnetic force (thrust) and torque (orientation) on the microrobot

configurations (Jin, 1999). For example, the Helmholtz coil configuration consists of two identical coils that are placed on the same axis and separated by a distance equal to the radius of the coils. This arrangement generates a uniform field close to the center of the coil pair when current passes in the same direction in both coils. A similar configuration called the Maxwell coil can generate a uniform gradient near the center. *Figure 14.4* shows a plot of the superimposed fields from Helmholtz and Maxwell coils. Both of these coil types are commonly used in MRI systems. The magnetic steering principle was demonstrated using a small scale system. The microrobot was put inside a plastic, maze-like structure with 1000 μm wide, water-filled channels. The maze was inserted at the center of a pair of concentric Maxwell and Helmholtz coils that were actuated to rotate around the maze. The current through the coils were regulated to control the force and torque (ie the forward thrust and orientation) on the robot independently. Numerous trials with the system confirmed that the independent orientation/thrust control principle was successful. Recent efforts at IRIS are towards applying this principle in a larger scale in combination with on-board magnetic actuators.

In conclusion, biomedical microrobotics is the next big challenge in the field of robotics. It combines the established theory and techniques of robotics (eg. motion control, path planning, remote operation or sensor fusion) with the exciting new tools enabled by MEMS technology to significantly improve the quality of our lives. The direction of international robotics research efforts are already shifting towards this direction. Effective collaboration between medical and robotics experts is an important key for the success of this technology of the future.

Key points for *Chapter 14*

- Biomedical microrobotics: Advanced mechatronic systems, positioned inside the body for medical diagnosis and intervention.
- Different sizes and designs for different target areas of the body.
- The gastrointestinal tract was the target area of first commercial applications.
- Energy storage and high degree of integration become the critical issues as the size goes down to sub-mm. MEMS technology becomes essential.
- Energy transfer with ex-vivo generated magnetic fields is a possible solution to this problem.
- Biomedical microrobotics may become a driving application for Hybrid MEMS technology.
- The volumetric-scaling of magnetic forces necessitate stronger and better controlled field sources than those commonly used in medical imaging.
- Coil systems for generating uniform magnetic field and field gradients can be employed to reduce the difficulties in control.
- Biomedical microrobotics is fast becoming one of the most active research fields in robotics.
- Effective collaboration between medical and robotics experts is needed.

References

Amblard F, Yurke B *et al* (2000) 'A Magnetic Manipulator for Studying Local Rheology and Micromechanical Properties of Biological Systems', *Rev Sci Instruments* **67(3):** 818–27

Dario P, Carrozza MC *et al* (1996) 'A Microrobot System for Lower Gastrointestinal Inspection and Intervention'. In: Di Natale C and D'Amico A (eds), *Sensors and Microsystems*: World Scientific Publishing Co Pte Ltd, Singapore 14–21

Grady MS, Howard MA III *et al* (1990) 'Nonlinear magnetic stereotaxis: Three-dimensional, *in vivo* remote magnetic manipulation of a small object in canine brain' *Med Phy* **17(3):** 405–15

Haber C, Wirtz D (2000) 'Magnetic Tweezers for DNA Micromanipulation' *Rev Sci Instruments* **7(12):** 4561–70

Hafeli U, Schutt W *et al* (1997) *Scientific and Clinical Applications of Magnetic Carriers,* Plenum New York

Holligan DL, Gilles GT *et al* (2003) 'Magnetic Guidance of Ferrofluidic Nanoparticles in an In Vitro Model of Intraocular Retinal Repair'. *IOP Nanotechnol* **14:** 661–6

Jin J (1999) *Electromagnetic Analysis and Design in Magnetic Resonance Imaging* CRC Press Florida

Kim B, Jeong Y *et al* (2003) Menciassi, P. Dario, Functional Colonoscope Robot System. Paper presented at the IEEE International Conference on Robotics and Automation (ICRA), Taipei, Taiwan: 14 September – 19 September

Mathieu JB, Martel S *et al* (2000) MRI Systems as a Mean of Propulsion for a Microdevice in Blood Vessels, IEEE International Conference on Engineering in Medicine and Biology

Sun Y, Potasek DP *et al* (2005) 'Characterizing Fruit Fly Flight Behavior Using a Microforce Sensor with a Novel Comb Drive Configuration'. IEEE/ASME *J Microelectromech Sys* **14(1):** 4–11

Vicci L (2001) A 3D Magnetic Force Manipulator DC Prototype, UNC Chapel Hill Dept. Of Computer Science Technical Report, no. TR01–031

www.givenimaging.com

www.rfnorika.com

www.stereotaxis.com

Yesin KB, Nelson BJ (2004) Robust CAD Model Based Visual Tracking for 3D Microassembly Using Image Space Potentials. Paper presented at the IEEE International Conference on Robotics and Automation (ICRA), New Orleans, US: 26 April – 01 May

Yesin KB, Vollmers K *et al* (2004) 'Analysis and Design of Wireless Magnetically Guided Microrobots in Body Fluids'. Paper presented at the IEEE International Conference on Robotics and Automation (ICRA), New Orleans, US: 26 April – 01 May

Zborowski M (1997) 'Physics of Magnetic Cell Sorting'. In: Hafeli, Schutt, Teller, Zborowski *et al*, *Scientific and Clinical Applications of Magnetic Carriers*, Plenum New York 205–32

CHAPTER 15

Nanotechnology and its applications in urology

IS Shergill, M Arya

Nanotechnology is the creation of functional material devices and systems through the control of matter on an atomic or molecular scale – the nanometer scale ($1nm = 10^{-9}m$). Preliminary designs of nanoparticles, such as artificial red blood cells, white cells and killer cells that can identify a particular bacteria, or cancer cells, have already been developed, and it is widely anticipated that nanotechnology will enable urologists to intervene at the cellular and molecular level of any disease process in the future.

In this chapter we introduce important concepts of nanotechnology and discuss published data in the urological literature that shows the potential for nanotechnology to link molecular signatures to urological cancer behaviour and clinical outcome, to develop nanoparticle probes for molecular and cellular imaging of urological disease and for the novel use of nanoparticles in the delivery of drug therapy.

Introduction

Imagine a world in which a miniscule chip can be used in the molecular genetics laboratory to accelerate research and to help identify markers of diagnostic, prognostic and therapeutic value. Imagine a world in which drugs can be delivered selectively to individual cells in the human body and thus treat potentially incurable diseases. Imagine a world in which robots are sent into the circulation with the mission of detecting cancer cells, disabling them and then causing their selective excretion through the kidneys. This is the world of nanotechnology, in which imagination is fast becoming a reality.

The prefix 'nano' comes from the Greek word *nanos*, which means 'little old' or 'dwarf'. By definition, nanotechnology is the study, design, creation, synthesis, manipulation and application of functional materials, devices and systems through control of matter at the nanometre scale. Nanomedicine is the monitoring, repair, construction and control of human biological systems at the molecular level, using engineered nanodevices and nanostructures. One nanometre is one billionth of a metre ($1nm = 10^{-9}m$), and it is at this size scale that most biological molecules inside living cells operate. For example, a DNA molecule is 2.5nm long and a sodium atom is about 0.2nm in size. Over the next decade it is widely expected that nanotechnology and nanomedicine will have important and innovative applications in clinical research and medicine, as well as contributing one trillion dollars to the global economy *(http://nsf.gov/eng/engadvise/PastMeetings/documents/nanoupdate_000.ppt).*

Potential applications of nanotechnology in urology

There are a wide range of potential applications of nanotechnology in the field of urology. This ranges from prevention of disease to early detection and improvements in diagnosis. In addition, treatment, prognosis, symptom management and drug delivery of many urological conditions can be accelerated with nanotechnological devices. In fact, nearly every use of nanotechnology and nanomedicine can have potential application in the field of urology.

Drug delivery systems and gene therapy

Delivery systems for drugs and gene therapy are particularly attractive targets in urological practice *(Figure 15.1)*. Novel drug delivery for prostate cancer using ceramic nanoparticles, carbon magnetic nanoparticles, protospheres and nanogold particles have been investigated in prostate cancer. Paclitaxel-loaded, biodegradable nanoparticles have been shown to be effective inhibitors of human prostate cancer cell lines in a murine model (Sahoo *et al*, 2004). In addition, enhanced cellular uptake of a triplex-forming oligonucleotide by nanoparticle formation in the presence of polypropylenimine dendrimers has also been found in metastatic prostate cancer cell lines, indicating their potential use for delivering therapeutic oligonucleotides in cancer cells in-vivo (Santhakumaran *et al*, 2004). Furthermore, Thomas *et al* (2004) have shown in-vitro targeting of synthesized antibody against prostate-specific membrane antigen with conjugated dendrimer nanoparticles as a suitable platform for targeted molecule delivery into appropriate antigen-expressing cells.

Studies investigating gene therapy in prostate cancer have also shown enhanced in-vitro DNA transfection efficiency by novel folate-linked nanoparticles (Hattori and Maitani, 2004), and similarly a human transferrin-targeted cationic liposome-DNA complex – transferring lipoplex – has shown enhanced stability, improved in-vivo gene transfer efficiency and long-term efficacy for systemic p53 gene therapy when used in combination with conventional radiotherapy (Xu *et al*, 2002).

Sawicki *et al* (Anderson *et al*, 2004) have demonstrated that a polymer, termed C32, is capable of delivering genes to cancer cells more efficiently and with less toxicity than other polymers that have been tested in the field to date. Therapeutic genes delivered to cells in this manner are able to drive cellular production of a gene-encoded protein through normal processes. By genetically engineering the normal diphtheria toxin gene, a toxin was created that would be produced only in prostate cells. When injected into prostate tumours in animals with C32 nanoparticles, tumor growth was suppressed or reversed, relative to untreated tumors.

Research is also being carried out to explore whether nanoparticles can be delivered intravenously to attack metastatic tumor cells, which are found throughout the body in advanced stages of cancer (*http://nanotechwire.com/news.asp?nid=1523*).

Nanotechnology and uroradiology

Body or organ imaging and labelling with nanostructure materials are also being used as adjuncts to uroradiological diagnosis. Recently, Harisinghani *et al* (2003) have demonstrated that highly lymphotropic super-paramagnetic nanoparticles, which gain access to lymph nodes by means of interstitial lymphatic fluid transport, enable the high-resolution magnetic resonance imaging of clinically occult lymph node metastases in patients with prostate cancer, which previously have not been detectable by any other non-invasive approach. It is inevitable that nano-uroradiology will be clinically useful in the future in uro-oncology (bladder, prostate and kidney cancer), as well as in non-cancer cases (urinary tract stones).

Nanotechnology and urological research

Basic science urological research has undoubtedly benefited from the advantages of nanotechnology, and in the future it is expected that not only will ongoing preclinical work be accelerated, but meaningful clinical studies using nanotechnology devices will be performed rapidly, with results and outcomes useful for clinical practice available as early as the next decade. Particular tools available for performing research include nanowires and nanotubes:

- Nanowires are sensing wires that can be coated with molecules to bind to proteins of interest and transmit their information through electrodes to computers.

- Nanotubes are cylinder-like assemblies of carbon atoms with cross-sectional dimensions in the nanometre range, and lengths that can extend over a thousand times their diameter.

Using such devices, several thousand sensors can be placed on a single chip, offering even greater multiplexing advantages. A variety of novel devices are emerging, such as microarrays with their high-precision patterning of biological molecules, useful for molecular diagnostics, genotyping and biomarker-guided therapeutic targeting (Ferrari, 2005).

Nanotechnology and prostate-specific antigen

Nanocantilevers are flexible beams, resembling a row of diving boards that can be coated with molecules capable of binding biomarkers. Using such nanotechnology, Wu *et al* (2001) demonstrated the quantification of prostate-specific antigen (PSA) at clinically significant concentrations. In addition, a novel reagent for low-level detection in immunoadsorbent assays has been described by Grubisha *et al* (2003). The reagent consists of gold nanoparticles modified to integrate bioselective species, such as antibodies, with molecular labels for the generation of intense, biolyte-selective, surface-enhanced Raman scattering (SERS) responses in immunoassays and other bioanalytical applications. In this study Grubisha *et al* demonstrated free PSA levels of approximately 1pg/ml in human serum.

Nanotechnology and treatment

Nanoshells, which are gold shell nanoparticles surrounded by a semiconductor that can be heated resulting in irradiation of the target cell, have been recently used to eradicate transmissible venereal tumours in mice (Hirsch *et al*, 2003). It is widely anticipated that nanoshells will be of widespread use in many urological cancers in the future.

Although further applications of nanotechnology in urology are less well advanced, arguably they have potentially significant implications. Surgical tools, such as nanotweezers are already in development, and it is anticipated that their everyday use in microsurgical procedures, such as vasectomy reversal and varicocoele repair, are only a few years away. In addition, nanoprobes aiding diagnostic procedures, such as 'nanourobots' used for cystoscopy, ureterosocpy and fulguration of tumours, as well as searching the inferior vena cava and renal vein to detect venous involvement of renal cell cancer, may be just around the corner (*Figure 15.2*). Smart nanosensors with communication capability and synthetic therapeutic devices to provide minimally invasive therapies will undoubtedly be developed, with particular interest in urological tissue engineering for urinary tract reconstruction (Shergill *et al*, 2006).

Nanotechnology and limitations

There are potential problems associated with nanotechnology that will have to be fully addressed before universal acceptance. The time required for ascertaining their suitability for clinical use might therefore be quite substantial, but it appears that the establishment of faster, safe regulatory approval protocols would ameliorate concerns about the length of time it takes for agents to be assessed (Ferrari, 2005). Ethical, socio-economic, political and environmental concerns are real, and in addition there will be a requirement for stringent regulations to prevent potential misuse, such as for terrorist activities.

Nanotechnology and the future

The growing importance of nanotechnology is reflected by the increase in the US Federal nanotechnology budget, from $270 million in the financial year 2000 to $738 million in 2003 (*http://www.nano.gov/2003budget.html*). The National Institute of Health has awarded researchers grants totalling nearly $10 million to establish a multidisciplinary research programme in cancer nanotechnology and to develop a new class of nanoparticles for molecular and cellular imaging. Working at the subatomic level, these scientists will be seeking data that will link molecular signatures to patients' clinical outcomes, so that cancers can be predicted, detected earlier and treated more effectively. The primary focus of the new programme will be prostate cancer.

Conclusions

Nanotechology is expected to have a significant impact on urological research and clinical practice, and will enable urologists to intervene at the cellular and molecular level, with diagnostic and therapeutic clinical benefit. A blockbuster movie based on Michael Crichton's (2002) nanotechnology bestseller *Prey* will be released shortly, further raising the profile of nanotechnology in the public domain.

Concepts such as nanovectors for targeted drug delivery, nanowires and nanocantilever arrays for the early detection of precancerous and malignant lesions, nanopores for DNA sequencing, and nanotubes and nanosensors for advanced delivery of therapeutic agents are quickly moving from imagination to a reality, with significant applications relevant to the diagnosis, management and treatment of all urological conditions.

Key points for *Chapter 15*

- Nanotechnology will have important and innovative applications in clinical research and medicine, as well as contributing one trillion dollars to the global economy.

- Novel drug delivery for prostate cancer using ceramic nanoparticles, carbon magnetic nanoparticles, protospheres and nanogold particles have been investigated in prostate cancer.

- Nanoprobes aiding diagnostic procedures are imminent.

- There are potential problems associated with nanotechnology that will have to be fully addressed before universal acceptance.

- Nanotechology is expected to have a significant impact on urological research and clinical practice, and will enable urologists to intervene at the cellular and molecular level, with diagnostic and therapeutic clinical benefit.

References

Anderson DG, Peng W *et al* (2004) A polymer library approach to suicide gene therapy for cancer. *Proc Natl Acad Sci USA;* **101(45):** 16028–33

Crichton M (2002) *Prey.* Harper Collins http://www.crichton-official.com/prey/index.html

Ferrari M (2005) Cancer nanotechnology: opportunities and challenges. *Nature Rev Cancer* **5:** 161–71

Grubisha DS *et al* (2003) Femtomolar detection of prostate-specific antigen: an immunoassay based on surface-enhanced Raman scattering and immunogold labels. *Anal Chem* **75(21):** 5936–43

Harisinghani MG *et al* (2003) Noninvasive detection of clinically occult lymph-node metastases in prostate cancer. *N Engl J Med* **348(25):** 2491–9

Hattori Y and Maitani Y (2004) Enhanced *in-vitro* DNA transfection efficiency by novel folate-linked nanoparticles in human prostate cancer and oral cancer. *J Control Release* **97:** 173–83

Hirsch LR *et al* (2003) Nanoshell-mediated near-infrared thermal therapy of tumours under magnetic resonance guidance. *Proc Natl Acad Sci USA* **100:** 13549–54

Sahoo SK, Ma W *et al* (2004) Efficacy of transferrin-conjugated paclitaxel-loaded nanoparticles in a murine model of prostate cancer. *Int J Cancer* **112(2):** 335–40

Santhakumaran LM, Thomas T *et al* (2004) Enhanced cellular uptake of a triplex-forming oligonucleotide by nanoparticle formation in the presence of polypropylenimine dendrimers. *Nucleic Acids Res* **32(7):** 2102–12

Shergill IS *et al* (2006) Nanotechnology: potential applications in urology. *Br J Urol Int* (in press) **97(2):** 219–20

Thomas TP *et al* (2004) *In-vitro* targeting of synthesized antibody-conjugated dendrimer nanoparticles. *Biomacromolecules* **5(6):** 2269–74

Wu G *et al* (2001) Bioassay of prostate-specific antigen (PSA) using microcantilevers. *Nat Biotechnol* **19(9):** 856–60

Xu L *et al* (2002) Self-assembly of a virus-mimicking nanostructure system for efficient tumour-targeted gene delivery. *Hum Gene Ther* **13(3):** 469–81

CHAPTER 16

Robotic surgery: the coming of a new era in surgical innovation

JV Joseph, HRH Patel

Introduction

There is hardly a surgical field where open procedures are not performed in a minimally invasive fashion, using 'keyhole' size openings to access the target organ. Whether simple or complex the majority of surgical procedures have been successfully performed or attempted laparoscopically. In a number of fields open surgery has been completely replaced by laparoscopy, such as cholecystectomy (NIH consensus statement, 1993). Similarly in urology open nephrectomies are being replaced by the laparoscopic approach (Joseph *et al*, 2003). Currently, there is a laparoscopic charge underway for several common procedures such as prostatectomy, cystectomy, cardiac valve surgery and revascularization surgeries, as well as others (Guillonneau and Vallancien, 2000; Rassweiler *et al*, 2003; Mamazza *et al*, 2001).

The success of laparoscopy has been due to its overall appeal to both patients and surgeons. The 'keyhole' sized openings used, resulted in shorter convalescence due to the overall reduction of trauma to the body. We have already advanced from using 10mm holes to access the target organ, to 5mm, and to instruments as small as 2mm ('needlescopic'), limiting the collateral trauma associated with surgical intervention (Cheah *et al*, 1998; Soper *et al*, 1994). Procedures that normally require a postoperative stay are now performed on an outpatient basis, with improved cosmesis (Hanly and Talamini, 2004). Patients require less post- operative care and recover faster; consequently returning to their normal routine more rapidly.

Traditional 'keyhole' surgery offers a number of advantages over the open approach; however several drawbacks limit its widespread adoption. These procedures performed laparoscopically are easier on the patient, but provide significant challenges to the surgeon. Conventional laparoscopic instrumentation offers poor ergonomics, limits a surgeon's range of motion, eliminates tactile feedback, and loses three dimensional visualization.

As technology has improved, these limitations are being addressed improving the surgeon's ability to perform complex procedures. The development of Robots to assist in surgeries has allowed a surgeon to regain range of motion, with increased precision and dexterity through tremor filtration and motion scaling. In addition, recent optical developments have allowed a three dimensional visualization lost with conventional laparoscopy (Camarillo *et al*, 2003). With robotic assistance, surgeons perform procedures in a minimally invasive fashion, with equivalent or even higher standards, compared to traditional open surgery.

Robots in surgery are not new. For the last twenty years or so, robots of different forms, performing a variety of functions have been used in the operating theatre (Marescaux *et al*, 2004). With the arrival of the daVinci™ robot over the last five years however, robot assisted surgery has been increasingly performed, leading many to question the future of open surgery in a number of surgical disciplines. In urology for example, the robot is transforming prostatectomy which has been known as a highly complex procedure in the open setting, and even more so with the laparoscopic approach. Similarly the precise suturing required for cardiac valve surgeries is being transformed by the robot as these procedures become more technically feasible.

Despite the steady improvements made in the use of robots in surgery, many surgeons continue to perceive the robot as a temporary phenomenon in the operating room. The reasons for this are varied, but include reservations about new technology. Robotic surgery however, is here to stay for several reasons: (1) patients seem to recover faster because the surgery causes less collateral damage; (2) the technology will get cheaper as competition in the market unfolds; and (3) the average surgeon using the robot will have access to becoming a master surgeon with robotic assistance. With continued innovation and technological improvement, the robot will continue to redefine how surgery is performed. It is a rather disruptive technology compared to the regular flow of open surgery. However it is steadily improving, increasingly meeting the needs of users. Robots have gone from a camera holding role, to one where they work as an extension of a surgeon's fingers. The technology is being shunned by most sophisticated laparoscopists who continue to develop their skills, which the robot may soon render obsolete. Emerging robotic technology is poised to cause disruption to both laparoscopists and open surgeons who will resist its adoption. It will continue to be a challenge to let go of what has been successful for decades, to put aside what has been perceived as the 'gold standard'.

The tepid reaction to the robot has been due to a number of factors. The daVinci robot for example has an initial cost of more than a million dollars, and maintenance cost approaching a quarter of a million dollars which prohibit its adoption at most medical centers around the world. It provides superb ergonomics, allowing the surgeon to perform complex procedures with ease. As it stands however, it is cumbersome, occupying a large space over the patient, making it difficult for the bedside assistant. Undoubtedly, robot manufacturers will eventually improve in this regard, improving robotic functionality and increasing miniaturization using technology that is already available. Next generation robots will need to augment the reality a surgeon already has. Sensory, haptic feedback is necessary for the robotic arms (not yet available) to be a true extension of a surgeon's finger tips. Similar to the improved 3-D visualization, improved high fidelity sensors will allow sensation beyond what is normally perceived with the human touch. Next generation surgical systems will allow the integration of all available data, and imaging studies to be used seamlessly to allow the surgeon to work, making microsurgical manipulation, while providing the utmost precision. Combination of live laparoscopic images, with virtual 3-dimensional images, reconstructed from 2mm sliced enhanced spiral computer tomography scanning, have been used to further aid in spatio-temporal awareness and allow proprioceptive feedback keys in laparoscopic surgery. Marescaux reported the first use of this technology in humans, performing a laparoscopic adrenalectomy. The reconstructed 3-D images helped identify, and avoid injury to the adrenal vein. This technique allowed increased delineation of dissection planes, and helped avoid injury to structures not directly in view of the laparoscope (Vogt 2003). In addition to reality augmentation, future robots will be equipped with sensors capable of detecting changes taking place as a result of tissue manipulation, or due to the stress associated with surgery. Advances in microelectrical mechanical systems (MEMS) will allow these to be a reality very soon.

It has taken a long time to go from large cumbersome surgical instruments to the current delicate ones allowing previously unknown surgical intervention. With the fast pace of present day technological improvements, microrobots are just around the corner. 'Keyhole' surgery is making large incisions a thing of the past. Will 'keyhole' itself be relegated to history in the near future, as part of what one can describe as natural surgical evolution? Abdominal exploration preceded the use of peritoneal lavage in the management of selected cases of blunt abdominal trauma. Laparoscopy, using trocars as small as 2mm, are used at some centers to evaluate patients in this setting. One can predict that soon the emergency room staff, or the ambulance personnel in the field will be able to place a microrobot in the form of a capsule inside a patient via a nasogatric tube, which will survey the bowel and other viscera to assess for possible injuries requiring surgical intervention. It may render diagnostic laparoscopy unnecessary, while it avoids the unfortunate delays which lead to the significantly high mortality seen in the early moments following an accident. Virtual capsule colonoscopy is a practical application of this concept currently in use (Lewis and Goldfarb, 2003; Jager *et al*, 2000). Will such a capsule be able to intervene, have the processing capability, using artificial intelligence applications to restore the integrity of affected or diseased structures?

A number of inventors have reported on the use of microrobots capable of intervening at the cellular level. Edwin W H Jager of Sweden's Linkoping University, recently reported experiments where robots (measuring 670 microns tall, 170–240 microns wide) were used to move tiny glass beads invisible to the naked eye (Jager *et al*, 2000) These robots can be made mobile, with arms, wrists, and fingers capable of carrying out defined tasks. They are capable of working submerged in liquids, such as urine, or blood, bypassing limitations of artificially flying insects, and silicon microrobots which could not operate under water. These microrobots can serve to both diagnose, and deliver necessary treatment at the cellular level, extending our capabilities to unimaginable levels. They will certainly redefine our notion of minimally invasive intervention. Will they have a preventative role, capable of correcting cellular damage, before the rest of the tissue or organ is affected, well before an abnormality became clinically significant? However we choose to use these microrobots, they will generate debates of similar magnitude to those currently generated by stem cell research applications.

In the current era whether a robot is used to augment the reality of the surgical field, or standard laparoscopic equipment is used, we are in awe when we compare 'keyhole' surgery to interventions where large incisions are made. Just as 'keyhole' surgery is steadily replacing open surgery, emerging technologies will also lead to the disruption of keyhole surgery, as more functional and reliable microrobots are developed. The immersive surgical experience provided by the available robots can be augmented further when all of a surgeon's senses are in use. One must be ready to assess available technologies in order to select the ones that promise the greatest good to the patients we serve. Keyhole surgery which is still in its infancy is filled with promises and surprises, as unexpected utilization or abandonment are recognized. Proper collaboration is necessary among surgeons, biomedical engineers, equipment manufacturers, health care administrators, and ethicists to speed the course of surgical evolution, improving outcome while we hold our promise to do no harm. Only with such an approach will we limit the ethical concerns raised by Asimov as we actively gather more autonomous, and intelligent tools in our armamentarium (Asimov, 1982).

Key points for *Chapter 16*

- Miniaturization of robots is becoming a reality.

- 3-dimensional reconstructive imaging allows virtual anatomical reconstruction of individual patients, aiding surgeons in planning the operation.

- Robots are here to stay, and will evolve to aid in many areas of medicine.

References

Asimov I (1982) *The Complete Robot*, Doubleday, Garden City, NY

Camarillo DB, Krummel TM (2004) Robotic Technology in Surgery: Past, Present, Future. *Am J Surg* **188:** 2–12

Cheah WK, Goh P *et al* (1998) So J Needlescopic retrograde cholecystectomy. *Surg Laparosc Endosc* **8:** 237–8

Guillonneau B, Vallancien G (2000) Laparoscopic radical prostatectomy: the Montsouris experience. *J Urol* **163:** 418–22

Hanly EJ, Talamini MA (2004) Robotic Abdominal Surgery. *Am J Surg* **188:** 19S–26S

Jager EW, Inganas O *et al* (2000) Microrobots for micrometer-size objects in aqueous media: potential tools for single-cell manipulation. *Science* **288:** 2335–8

Joseph JV, Madeb R *et al* (2003) Laparoscopic Surgery in Urology: Nephrectomy and Prostatectomy. *Hosp Med* **64:** 441–5

Lewis B, Goldfarb (2003) The Advent of Capsule Endoscopy – a not so futuristic approach to obscure gastrointestinal bleeding *Aliment Pharmacol Ther* **17:** 1085–96

Mamazza J, Schlachta CM *et al* (2001) Needlescopic surgery. A logical evolution from conventional laparoscopic surgery. *Surg Endosc* **15:** 1208–12

Marescaux J, Rubino F *et al* (2004) Augmented-reality-assisted laparoscopic adrenalectomy. *J Am Med Ass* **292:** 2214–5

NIH (1993) NIH consensus statement: gallstones and laparoscopic cholecystectomy. *J Am Med Ass* **269:** 1018–24

Rassweiler J, Seemann O *et al* (2003) Laparoscopic versus open radical prostatectomy: a comparative study at a single institution. *J Urol* **169:** 1689–93

Soper NJ, Brunt LM *et al* (1994) Laparoscopic general surgery. *New Engl J Med* **330:** 409–19

Vogt W (2003) Imaging in gastroenterology – what is new? Schweizerische Rundschau fur *Medizin Praxis* **92:** 1435–41

Index

contact laser ablation of the prostate (CLAP)
37
cost–benefit ratio 96–7
cost-containment 94
costs *see* healthcare costs
cryoablation, renal cell carcinoma 54
cryosurgery, prostate cancer 44
Cushing syndrome 23–4
cutting balloon, hot-wire 52
cystocele 114
cystoscopes, historical development 1–2
cystoscopy
    nanourobots 146
    virtual 67

D

daVinci™ system 6, 125, 130–1, 132–3, 152
day case surgery, laparoscopic
    cholecystectomy 18
Decker, Albert 2
detrusor sphincter dyssynergia (DSD) 41, 42
dexterity 131
diagnostic general surgery 11–14
diaphragmatic injury 12
diverticular disease, colectomy 23
Dornier lithotripter 64, 65
drug delivery systems, nanotechnology 144–5
Dubois, François 3
dysphagia, anti-reflux syndrome 20–1

E

economics 93–8
efficacy evaluation 97
    benign prostatic hyperplasia *38*
endocrine surgery 23–5
EndoLoop applicator 3
endopyeloplasty, percutaneous 52
endopyelotomy, percutaneous 52
endoscopic retrograde
    cholangiopancreatography (ERCP)
    18, 20
endoscopic simulator 67
endoscopy

    history 1–3
    skill sets *85*
endoureterotomy 51
end-stage renal disease 103–4
epigastric artery, inferior, damage 73–4
ergonomic positioning 131
esophageal carcinoma 22–3
esophagectomy, sub-total 22–3
ethics
    organ donation 105–6
    robotics use 153
external beam radiotherapy (EBRT), prostate
    cancer 44
extracorporeal shockwave lithotripsy (ESWL)
    53

F

femoral hernia repair 25, 26
Fenger-plasty repair 52
fluoroscopy, real-time 67
fundoplication
    re-do 21
    see also Nissen fundoplication,
    laparoscopic

G

gall bladder carcinoma 18
gallstones
    laparoscopic cholangiography 19
    laparoscopic cholecystectomy 17–18
gas bloat syndrome 20
gas embolism 75–6
gastrectomy, total 22, 23
gastric arteries, short (SGA) 20, *21*
gastric banding 21–2
gastric carcinoma 22–3
gastric diversion 21
gastrointestinal cancers
    colorectal surgery 23
    esophageal carcinoma 22–3
    gastric carcinoma 22–3
    recurrence rate 23
    staging laparoscopy 14

W

Z

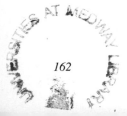